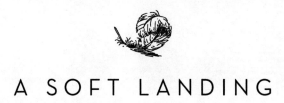

A SOFT LANDING

A Soft LANDING

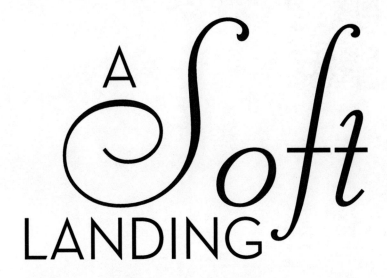

how ONE WOMAN *survived*
A COLLISION COURSE WITH *death*

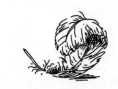

stacey BLAKE

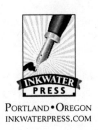

INKWATER PRESS

PORTLAND • OREGON
INKWATERPRESS.COM

*Scan this QR Code
to learn more about
this title*

Cover and interior design by Masha Shubin
Cover images (source: Bigstockphoto.com): A human figure walking © Sergey
Nivens; Flying white feather © viperagp; Tear paper abstract © Petr Vaclavek;
Vector damask © Kathryn Stitt. Internal: Hand drawn feathers © canicula.

Paperback ISBN-13 978-1-62901-014-4 | ISBN-10 1-62901-014-6
Kindle ISBN-13 978-1-62901-015-1 | ISBN-10 1-62901-015-4

Printed in the U.S.A.
All paper is acid free and meets all ANSI standards for archival quality paper.

1 3 5 7 9 10 8 6 4 2

With deepest love to my wonderful brother Tim

Table of Contents

Acknowledgments ix

Listen to Your Body xiii

Foreword xv

Prologue xxv

Ch. 1: How It Began 1

Ch. 2: The Beginnings: How I First Met God 17

Ch. 3: The Struggle to Understand the "Why" of My Illness 32

Ch. 4: The Divine Experience That Changed My Life Forever... 42

Ch. 5: More Miracles 65

Ch. 6: Tom at My Side – My Stem Cell Transplantation 77

Ch. 7: Faith Everlasting 87

Ch. 8: A Medical Setback 101

Ch. 9: Releasing the Past 111

Ch. 10: Love Heals All...127

Epilogue 134

Michael 138

I Promise 140

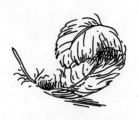

Acknowledgments

S O MUCH OF THIS BOOK IS A DIRECT RESULT OF DEEP PRAYER and long hours of quiet contemplation. I owe much to the Almighty for everything in my life. So of course, my highest appreciation for the gifts given to me rests in God.

Throughout my years, there have been a handful of friends that I have been able to count on during both good times and bad, but without exception my greatest loves in life have been my husband Tom and my stepchildren Christina and Jeffrey. They are the foundation for my life and I love them beyond words. As well, my incredibly loving mother and father-in-law Maribel and Bill. Thank you for always being with me in spirit through my difficult trials, your prayers of healing with me in all ways. My own mother, Virginia, thank you for every good lesson you taught me in my life. I am my mother's daughter in every way.

True friendships take years to bloom and be tested. I have within my heart a special place for those whose trust and confidence in me runs deep and true. My good friend and personal attorney Paul Kfoury, whom I have known since I was in college, my friend Ben, who has been a sincere friend since high school, as well my best friend Kathy, who is without equal in her devotion and unconditional support. Each one of my brothers has been a true friend along the journey of my life and I love each of them with all my heart. Always too, thank you, Michelle, for your cards and love during my recovery.

One of the greatest surprises my illness showed me was that I was loved by many more people than I realized. From my employees to my neighbors, who asked after me constantly, to the many acquaintances I had made in town through charity work and local affairs. Words of support and well wishes reached me every day. But most especially I was held close in the hearts of all of my family members at the 157th Air Refueling Wing and the 64th Air Force Refueling Squadron at Peace Air Base where Tom became stationed for three years as Chief Pilot in early 2010. He had been in the Air National Guard for many years while flying with US Airways and we knew everyone very well. There was not a day that went by when Tom did not come home and tell me that Father Bob or Z or Colonel Paul Hutchinson, Chan, Jimmy Doyle, Nelson Perron, and Nelson Abreu were asking about me and sending me love and words of support. Thank you to everyone who took care of and helped Tom through many difficult and dark days. Especially I wish to give personal thanks to Bonnie Rice and all of the members of the family readiness staff who cared for me when Tom needed to deploy. I love you all very much.

During my business career I have fond memories of several people who were exceptionally good individuals to know and work with, who provided me and my company opportunities to thrive. Rico Pastorino, Alan Hawkins, and Michael Leary, thank you each. I wish to acknowledge Bob Stanger, who was a true friend in so many ways as well as a solid private banking coordinator.

No acknowledgement would be complete for me without recognition of my oncology staff at Dana Farber, headed by my own Doctor – Dr. Joseph Antin. Dr. Antin provided me at all times throughout my difficult trials and recovery with a strong sense of confidence that I would be okay and all in time would be well. Priceless. All of my floor nurses were exceptional in their skills and knowledge. When my body was exhausted and spent, these incredible professionals gave me hope and strength each day.

My new editor Linda Franklin and the entire team at Inkwater Press have impressed me with their professionalism, rapid and thorough responses and supportiveness in all things related to helping me get this, my first book, completed.

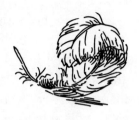

Listen to Your Body

M Y STORY IS ONE OF MANY PERSONAL SUCCESSES AND CHAL-
lenges, but one very important piece of advice that
I have for everyone is to listen to your body's silent
signals that it will give you when something inside … is
going wrong. The body is an amazing marvelous machine
in many respects and it will try in odd ways to alert and
warn you when "something" is going wrong deep inside.

Around the summer of 2008 I began to suffer episodes
of paranoia that seemed at the time to come out of nowhere,
plaguing me with intense feelings of fear that an imminent
crisis of some kind was about to occur. It manifested for
me in several ways. I had an Armageddon sense of doom
that there would be a major weather disaster in our area,
and to prepare for that I began to buy loads of dry goods,
forcing my husband Tom to build for me extra shelves for
all the canned goods and dried foods I was buying. On
a beautiful day by the pool in the summers of 2007 and
2008 I would suddenly be affected by intense feelings of
fear that an attack on the house by some dark "something"

was about to happen and (quite honestly) I was forced several times to seek refuge inside my bedroom closet, where I would hide for hours. Imagine how I saw myself inside my closet while hiding. Here I was a successful businesswoman, whose company had for over twenty-five years grossed upwards of $100 million in sales, confidence inside me abounding – here I was hiding in fear of some unknown bogeyman – in my bedroom closet on a beautiful sunny summer day.

Today, I have come to believe that these impulsive feelings of fear were my body's attempt to warn me that "something on the inside of me" was going wrong. That illness ... was taking hold of me and I was becoming sick. Had I tuned into that more accurately I probably could have caught my leukemia at a much earlier stage.

For anyone who has suffered unexpected and bizarre fears, without any real basis in reality – please consider asking your doctor to do a complete physical exam with blood work.

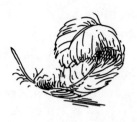

Foreword

"ND SO BEGAN THE BEGINNING OF THE END OF MY LIFE AS I had known it." In her autobiographical, gently told tale of her experience as a patient with leukemia, Stacey Blake makes this reality clear for the reader. She recounts the day of her leukemia diagnosis with absolute clarity. Then, she weaves her "other life story" into this one: her pre-leukemia story, making the contrast between the two all the more stark. For most, the trip to the doctor is motivated by vague complaints such as abdominal pain or fullness, bruising, or fatigue. Stacey describes herself feeling "as though the air was being let out of a balloon." Imagine: what you think will be a routine trip to the clinic turning into an urgent hospitalization and the beginning of a medical odyssey for which you have had no experience that could have prepared you. So begins Stacey's tale.

As a nurse working in the field of stem cell transplantation for nearly twenty years, I have been present with and witness to countless patients who have learned that they need stem cell transplantation. There is no way to prepare oneself for the conversation that follows such a revelation. The survival "numbers" are always shocking. Zero percent chance of survival without transplantation. Forty percent chance of long-term survival with the transplant, which is the only curative option. There are costs, though, associated with survival: loss of fertility, loss of sexual function, loss of income and a sense of competence, loss of the sense of being a contributing member of one's family, which can be replaced by the feeling of being a burden.

The reality that one could die from leukemia is made abundantly clear and yet treatment options seem daunting: chemotherapy, radiation, bone marrow transplant? For most, the issue of survival trumps the other losses in making the decision to move forward.

While bone marrow transplant can provide the life-saving option that leukemia patients hope for, it is dangerous and it can be painful. Infection is a serious concern as the patient's immune system is wiped out with chemotherapy. The new donor's immune system takes a long time to recover. For most, the immune function is still not normal even after the first year. The side effects associated with the chemotherapy and the radiation can be severe. At Dana Farber Cancer Institute we often acknowledge the difficulty with informed consent as there is no way that one can conceive of what lethal dose radiation can do to your body. Mouth sores sound manageable, but the reality of your gastrointestinal tract sloughing off and bleeding is something unimaginable.

When someone is diagnosed with a life-threatening disease such as leukemia, that reality can never be undone. Before these words are spoken, one would never imagine them. In the moments before the leukemia diagnosis is acknowledged, your symptoms are due to overwork, too much stress, a cold or flu: something one can easily recover from or fix. After, there is shock and disbelief. And there is trauma. What was once never part of your reality is forever more possible. I have seen patients for years after their transplants hold their breath until they receive the results of their blood counts and until they hear their doctor tell them, "Things are good. No signs of the leukemia." I have had other patients tell me that even years later, they still throw up before coming to their follow-up appointment. That is trauma.

Leukemia was first described in 1845 by Dr. Rudolf Virchow of Germany. He admitted Mary Straide, a fifty-year-old cook, to the hospital with complaints of swelling in her lower extremities and a cough that had persisted over the past year.[*] During the next three months, Mary's symptoms progressed. She experienced severe episodes of epistaxis, or nose bleeding and developed infectious blisters over the palms of her hands. Three months after her admission to the hospital, she passed away. Her autopsy revealed blood vessels that were filled with white, barely red blood that appeared more like pus. Initially, Virchow and his colleagues referred to this disease as "white blood." The overabundance of white blood cells made the blood look like pus, and most physicians of the day thought it to be an overwhelming infection or purulence of the blood. Virchow, however, understood that this was not the result of an infection but it was a disease of the white blood cells

---

[*] Seufert, W., & Seufert, W. (1982). The recognition of leukemia as a systemic disease. *Journal of the History of Medicine and Allied Sciences*, *37*(1), 34–50.

themselves. He recognized it as a neoplastic disorder, or a cancer of the blood, and he called it leukemia.

Cancer is, by definition, disordered cell growth. Blood cancers are characterized by disordered growth of the white blood cells, which fail to mature and function normally. As the leukemia cells proliferate, the abnormal cells crowd out the healthy ones, interfering with their function. It is this lack of normal cell function which is so dangerous to patients with leukemia. Untreated, the disease will progress, with the primary causes of death being infection due to lack of functional white blood cells or hemorrhage from lack of blood clotting platelets.

"How in the world did I get leukemia?" Newly diagnosed patients may point to all of the healthy habits that have shaped their lives. They may acknowledge the stress of their work and home lives and wonder whether these might have caused their illness. Some even consider the idea that they are being punished for something. There is an attempt to understand how this could happen, what one might have done to bring it on. If one can rationalize its occurrence, then perhaps, it can be undone? All of the cells in our bodies have the potential to undergo random genetic aberrations. In fact, we accumulate these mutations as we age. Leukemia is understood by science to be a result of these mutations. The leukemia cell is able to grow when this mutation does not repair itself or isn't able to turn itself off. While there are some clear associations between exposure to hazardous substances and the development of blood cancers, these cases are rare. For most, it is an inexplicable accident at the cellular level.

Stacey was diagnosed with chronic myeloid leukemia, or CML, in an accelerated phase. CML is characterized by a high white blood count and splenomegaly, or severe enlargement of the spleen. The bone marrow of CML patients may show evidence of the translocation of chromosomes 9 and 22, the genetic aberration that characterizes this particular leukemia. These two chromosomes break and then repair themselves incorrectly, combining with each other instead of their own chromosomes. When such patients are "blasting," or displaying blasts, immature cells, the disease can be transitioning to a more aggressive form or to acute leukemia.

Fortunately for Stacey, the treatment of this disease has evolved since Virchow first described it in the mid-1800s.[*] The first documented attempt at treating CML was with the use of arsenic in 1865. Administered in small doses, arsenic would decrease the white blood count. Unfortunately, it did not extend the life of the patient. Radiation became the standard therapy for nearly fifty years, beginning in the early 1900s. Radiation to the spleen improved symptoms, but again, it did not prolong the course of the disease. The earliest chemotherapy was developed around the time of World War II. Busulfan was an oral chemotherapy agent that could easily be taken and it was superior to the earlier treatments in controlling the blood counts, but there was no evidence that it improved survival or affected the progression of the disease. It was replaced by the drug Hydroxyurea in the 1970s, which was associated with fewer side effects and better control of the counts. This oral chemotherapy drug also provided the first modest effect on prolongation of survival of patients with CML.

---

[*]   Deininger, M. (2008). Chronic myeloid leukemia: An historical perspective.

Interferon was introduced as a treatment option in the early 1980s. It was the first drug that had the potential to induce a complete remission, which it did in a minority of cases. In those that did not achieve a remission, it had the potential to prolong the course of the disease and increase survival time. Unfortunately for many, the symptoms associated with taking Interferon were intolerable: fatigue, depression, fevers, and weight loss. It was like having an ongoing case of the flu.

Allogeneic stem cell or bone marrow transplant is the process of administering chemotherapy and/or radiation to reduce or eliminate the bone marrow stem cells and then infuse donor bone marrow stem cells into a patient with a disease such as leukemia. The first successful transplants were done in the late 1960s on children with immunologic diseases.[*] In 1977, 100 patients were treated with chemotherapy and radiation before receiving bone marrow from matched sibling donors. Just thirteen of them survived. Outcomes improved in the 1980s from roughly 15% survival to around 30% survival by the end of the decade. In 1987 The National Marrow Donor Program was founded so that the 70% of patients without matched related donors could have bone marrow transplants using matched unrelated donors. There have been more than 50,000 unrelated donor transplants done since that time.

By the end of the 1980s, more transplants were being done using related and unrelated donors. Mortality rates, though, were high. Infection, organ injury (liver, kidneys, and lungs), and graft versus host disease (GVHD), an

---

[*] Appelbaum, F., Forman, S., Negrin, R., & Blume, K. (Eds.). (2004). *Thomas' hematopoietic cell transplantation.*

immunological complication where the donor's immune system attacks the healthy tissue of the patient, were the life-limiting complications and unrelated donor transplants were riskier. Over the next two decades, the international transplant community worked towards making transplant safer and towards reducing complications such as GVHD, which limits the quality of the transplant survivor's life as well as his or her long-term survival. In a study comparing transplant outcomes between 1993–1997 and 2003–2007, risk of death from complications was reduced by more than 50%.* Having been in this field during that period of time, I am rewarded by seeing patients like Stacey recover not only from her transplant, but from the life-threatening complications that followed.

The discovery of imatinib or Gleevec in 1998, a tyrosine kinase inhibitor (TKI) that targets the specific protein that allows the CML cell to grow, has revolutionized the treatment of CML.** It has rendered transplant unnecessary for 95% of these patients with this form of leukemia, as it can induce a long-lasting remission with relatively few side effects. Whereas the average life expectancy before TKIs was just three to six years without a potentially dangerous transplant, these drugs produce a survival rate of 90% at ten years. The downside is that they control the disease rather than curing it, much like insulin does for diabetes. Therefore, patients need to continue taking the drugs, probably lifelong. Since the drugs are very expensive, costing

---

* Bortin, M.M., et al. (1992). Changing trends for allogeneic bone marrow transplantation for leukemia in the 1980's. *Jama, 5*(268), 607–12.

** Kantarjian, H., MD Anderson Cancer Center (2011). *TKI treatment for chronic myeloid leukemia.* 7/14/2011 [video/DVD] ecancer.tv.

approximately $90K/year at this time, for some this treatment is prohibitive. Insurance co-pays can be extremely high and some patients may stop taking it and the disease can relapse and progress.

In addition, Gleevec is not totally effective for some 5% of patients, who will then need a transplant. One cannot comprehend the effects of this process on their body through description. It is only through experiencing it that you begin to understand. Some patients have told me in the aftermath of this experience that they would not have chosen to move forward, had they known. Others are simply happy to have their lives extended with their loved ones, in spite of their differences. To have the chance to watch your children grow, to sit quietly with your husband, to experience the gift of the beauty the world has to offer, is enough. Some are very thankful but also are resentful of the changes in their bodies. This conflict of feelings can be difficult to reconcile.

As she tells her remarkable story, Stacey shares with us how she gets through this experience. She describes her unique experiences that led her into a strong foundation of faith and spirituality. She also is awed by the dedicated care of her family as she describes how they cared for her. It is imperative to have a supportive caretaker and for that caretaker to have support as well. Having someone with you who cares about you is one of the determinants of survival.

Stacey's transplant physician, Dr. Joseph Antin, began working in the field of transplantation in 1984. He has been one of the leaders in the field and has contributed to the advances that led to the reduction in mortality during the past twenty-nine years. His early work included allogeneic bone marrow transplant for patients with CML and he helped develop the concept and practice of donor lymphocyte infusions, or the infusion of donor T-cells which are immune cells, for the treatment of relapsed CML after transplantation. He is considered an expert in the treatment of GVHD and has led the research in that field as well.

It is extremely important for patients to have confidence in their physician. Their survival depends on it. There are many rules related to isolation or "the precautions" that one must take to protect themselves from infection, including no pets, no public places, no work, etc., and patients must understand that without heeding these restrictions, survival is impossible. Patients must buy into the process.

In my work as a transplant nurse, I have found that the relationship that I form with a patient is the basis for all of the work that follows. It is the stepping stone from which all interactions begin and where assessment and treatment of the patient's physical and emotional health occurs. In the eloquent words of Grayce Sills, a remarkable nurse and educator, "Anyone who has experienced one of these many human crises knows how helpful it is to have a guide and companion along the journey. However, if one is fortunate enough to have a skilled guide, informed by the intellect and empowered by competent caring, then one has been more than lucky. One has been blessed."

It is my honor to have been on this difficult journey with Stacey and the hundreds of other transplant patients that I have helped care for. The connection between Stacey's story and my role in her care is a spiritual one. It is the human connection that makes this so. For when you meet someone without prejudice or bias and with love, no matter whether there are vast differences in your life experiences, then that is a blessed interaction.

Toni Dubeau, RN.

Stem Cell Transplant Program Nurse,
Dana Farber Cancer Institute

Toni guides each patient and their family through the pretransplant process, answering questions, working with the team to move them to transplant, and providing comprehensive education to the patient and their support system. After the hospital discharge, her work with patients continues as she follows them for complications and provides answers to questions as they come along. When patients are sick and require care and rapid intervention, she is able to help facilitate that process.

ADDITIONAL BIBLIOGRAPHY

Beutler, E. (2001). The treatment of acute leukemia: past, present and future. *Leukemia, 15,* 658.

Goldman, J. (2010). History of chronic leukemia. *Seminars in Hematology, 47*(4), 302–311.

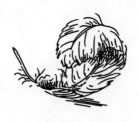

Prologue

"YOU HAVE LEUKEMIA, STACEY, AND YOU ARE VERY SICK. WE have no idea really how it is you even walked into this hospital," the doctor whom I had just met moments ago gently told me. In those five seconds my world changed forever.

How does one prepare for this kind of shock in one's life? You might have all the self-help books on the market, and try as you might to visualize the what-ifs in life, nothing, absolutely nothing, can prepare you for a diagnosis of leukemia or any other life-threatening illness, unless you have in your life a strength, an inner resource to guide you. You can have done yoga and meditation, you could have attended numerous in-vogue seminars on life and self-improvement, but without faith ... a true, deep, abiding, unshakeable faith in the goodness of life and in God, no matter what you may call him ... the pathway through the hells of illness and disease cannot be won, without "HIM" by your side.

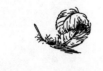

A SOFT LANDING

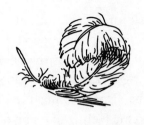

CHAPTER 1

How It Began

"TOM, I AM NOT FEELING VERY WELL," I SAID, CALLING HOME to my husband from my San Francisco Bay Area hotel room. "I think I would like to head out into the country for a weekend at a B&B to try to get some rest. I've been really tired this week, and I am coughing a lot. I don't feel ready to fly back to the East Coast just yet. I think I need a brief rest."

Tom said, "Sure, honey, are you sick?"

"I don't know? I don't think so … maybe just overtired. All this week I've been coughing. During my meeting at Safeway and all throughout lunch with the buyer, I had a persistent dry cough. Not a cold, but a cough. And between appointments, I needed to head back to my hotel room, to nap and recover some energy. I'm just really tired."

And so began the beginning of the end of my life as I had known it. Unbeknownst to me at that time, my life in a matter of days would change. It was June 2009, and during my weekend in the country, I could not walk two blocks without having to sit for long periods of rest. My sleep, while long, was not refreshing, and in general, I simply did not feel well. I could not say with any positive sense what was wrong. "I" though was not right. I was not feeling like myself.

As I drove to the airport to head home a few days later, I can recall the extreme feeling of being off balance with the car, while taking a long, wide exit ramp. I had a dizziness that felt like much more than typical vertigo, and I had to hold on tight, **tight** to the wheel, and **focus**, for fear that I would pass out and lose control of the car.

Once home, on that Tuesday, I called my mom and told her what I had been experiencing. Listening to me cough lightly all through the call, my mom asked me repeatedly to call my doctor for an appointment. I kept saying to her that all I needed was another day of solid rest. Mom persisted and repeated my need to call. Reluctantly, I agreed. Mom being Mom, before hanging up, asked that I do it the minute I hung up with her.

As I dialed my primary doctor's telephone number, at the Lahey Clinic in Burlington, Massachusetts, I almost stopped, thinking that really all I did need was another good day of quiet rest. The phone, however, was quickly answered and the nurse I was talking with said immediately, "Stacey, you need to come in to see us this week."

I told her, "I can't do that; I leave Thursday for Philadelphia."

"You are not going to Philadelphia on Thursday," she said. "You will be coming here tomorrow."

"But I have a presentation!"

She said, "We will need to see you first, and then see."

Within minutes my appointment for the next day was scheduled. I hung up thinking, *Wow; this is kind of a bit much, this whole thing.* Needing to go to the doctor's on such short notice, it felt to me almost like an over-reaction. Little did I know how wrong I had been ...

The next day began with a series of chest x-rays, blood work, breathing tests, and a visit to my primary physician. While traveling from one test to the other, I was exhausted. Several times I was so slow in my walking I thought I would just stop in the middle of the clinic's hallway. I could not understand what was wrong with me. It was as if air was being let out a balloon. I was fading by the minute. Finally, while I sat in the waiting room, the minutes ticked by. My appointment, which was to be at 11:00 AM, was delayed. Ten minutes, twenty minutes, then thirty minutes passed until a young nurse came out and said more time would be needed, and to not leave *or go anywhere,* but to wait. I nodded "ok."

I started to get the sense something odd was going to happen and I noticed that a few of the doctors inside the inner office were taking long looks at me, where I was sitting. A few of them appeared to be gaping at me. Peering back at them, I can remember not being able to shake the feeling that something seemed off. I tried to watch the TV, which was at the end of the room, but I could not focus. I had become aware that this visit seemed and felt different.

After a few more minutes, I was escorted into one of the small examining rooms by a nurse, where I met for the first time my new primary physician. She was an attractive young woman who appeared to me to be in her early thirties. She took a few minutes before addressing me. And while she took her time in starting, I noticed that the lights in this examining room seemed a bit dimmer than normal.

She began by asking me to review with her the symptoms

that brought me in that day. As I finished, she started to say, "You *have* ... uh, you *are* ... " She cleared her throat a little and stopped. She tried to speak again, but instead stopped. She looked down for moment, then up at me with genuine sadness and the beginnings of tears in her eyes. She said, "Please excuse me for a moment," and she quickly left the room.

Right outside the room I could see another doctor, a very tall male doctor with thick curly black hair who I had noticed looking at me earlier. He nodded to my primary and touched her arm in a reassuring manner before coming into the exam room. Immediately he stretched out his hand and shook mine, introducing himself as the Department head. He then asked, "Stacey, can you please explain again the symptoms you have had?"

I told him about the fact I had been experiencing a dry persistent cough, but also ... "yes, I had been having for a long time severe night sweats, trouble with bruising [adding with a laugh, that if you look at me the wrong way, I would develop a bruise somewhere on my body], and ... *come to think of it* ... yes, I have been having other unusual symptoms like dizziness, and feelings of fatigue, but I just figured that was because I work so many hours."

The doctor looked at me for a moment and then said very quietly, "You have leukemia, Stacey."

I replied with some puzzlement, *"I have what?"*

He said again, "You have been diagnosed with leukemia."

I waited a few seconds and asked, "Are you sure?"

"There is no mistake," he said.

I asked, "How do you know?"

"Your blood tests; your results have come back and your white blood count is 536,000."

I asked then, "And that is bad?"

He said, "Most definitely. Normal white blood counts should be around 5,000 or so. Yours are way too high."

I asked cautiously, "Could it be anything else?"

He said, "No, it is a certainty ... *there can be no other diagnosis.* We have retested your blood three times to be sure. You have **leukemia.** You are very sick, and we have no idea really how it is you even walked into this hospital. Yours is the highest white blood count we have seen, and you will not be walking anywhere further. We are bringing a wheelchair for you now, and at this time the front desk is preparing for you to be admitted into the hospital."

I was speechless. I was almost numb. I did not know what to say. My mind, having been trained throughout my business career to troubleshoot problems without drama, but with a certain precision, did not know at all what to say. I just sat there and tried to think of anything that might actually be incorrect in his diagnosis. It seemed impossible. I had never thought that anything like this could happen to me. So, I simply stared at this very nice man, who obviously did not like having to tell me any of this, and asked, "Can you cure me?"

"Maybe," he said, "*maybe.* Right now, Dr. Steinberg is being called to examine you in your room immediately after you arrive there." He looked down at the paperwork he had in front of him and asked, "You are married, is that right, Stacey?"

"Yes, I am."

He explained, "You need to call your husband and tell him to get down here immediately. Tell him to go straight into the Lahey Hospital, not the clinic, and tell him that you will be admitted into a room shortly. *Please,* do not tell him you have leukemia. Just ask him to get here as fast as possible."

I sat back, looked at the doctor, and said, "Okay, but ... "

He interrupted me, saying, "Trust me; just tell him to get down here quickly." As he got up to leave, the doctor sat back down for a few seconds and took a long look at me with what appeared to be a little hesitation, as if he was waiting for me to possibly break down, or cry, or to ask more questions. When I did not, he politely excused himself and left the room, leaving a nurse only a few feet away. It was then that I realized they really did think I just might keel over at any second. My mind though, as was my habit, was already compartmentalizing all of this new information, as I normally do with any sudden crisis within the company. Not yet did I comprehend *that this was personal!* **This was about me!** It was not about the company, like a small irritating delivery issue or a supply issue or a product issue, or anything that quickly could be fixed with a soothing phone call and a correct logistical hand. No, at this moment, I had no appreciation yet as to what was happening to me or what was to come.

After a few minutes, a nurse came back into the room and asked that I provide again my insurance card for the hospital admission. In a slight fog, I reached into my purse and got it for her, grabbing for my cell at the same time. I waited until she left the room and closed the door before calling my husband's work number. At the time, Tom was a pilot for US Airways, but he also worked part time for FlightSafety as a simulator instructor pilot. I had never had to place an emergency call in to Tom while he was at work, and as I dialed the number slowly, my hand began to shake.

Pete answered the phone.

"Pete, it's Stacey ... can you please find Tom for me right away?"

He replied, "He's in the simulator."

"This is an emergency, Pete; can you please get him for me immediately?"

"Yes, of course, Stacey; I'll get him for you right away."

It took several long minutes to get Tom, as the whole simulator needed to be shut down, and then Tom needed to be called on the phone inside where he was training. Not a small or inexpensive thing to do. About five minutes later, I heard Tom's voice, which since meeting him nearly seven years earlier, had always brought me immediate comfort. He asked, "What is it, honey?"

I replied with dead calm, "Tom, I am being admitted into the hospital right now at Lahey, and you need to get down here immediately."

"Are you injured?" Tom immediately asked.

"No, but please ... just get down here right away. I will talk to you when you get here, but right now a nurse is signaling to me that they are taking me to my room."

Being the flyboy that my husband is, Tom's reply was his signature for important things: "**ROGER THAT ... I AM ON IT!**"

Once in my room, I met a very special man, Dr. Steinberg. He was the head of Oncology at Lahey.

With his elegant but firm style, he came over to my bed and said, "Young lady, you are extremely sick ... and I need to determine quickly what kind of leukemia you actually have. To do that, I need to do a bone marrow biopsy. Now, I am going to be honest here, this is not going to be fun, but I need to do it and there is no time to lose, so we are going to do it right here in this bed. Are you okay with that?"

I asked, smiling, "Well, do I have a choice?"

Dr. Steinberg replied with a wink, "Well, actually no ... but it is always good to ask."

I liked Dr. Steinberg immediately. I felt he and I were going to get along just fine. I myself am very direct, but with a soft edge in my business dealings (unless I am crossed); with his kind eyes and straightforward manner, I relaxed.

Within about twenty minutes, Dr. Steinberg and his nurse came back into the room and with swift efficiency put me on my front, face down on the bed, explaining in near musical terms the process for the biopsy. While Dr. Steinberg was preparing the anesthetic needle, which did sting slightly when given, little did I realize what was to come next with this procedure. All my life, I have dreaded needles and the taking of blood. I'd had some experience with needles, due to a hospital stay for three weeks in 2001, but nothing had prepared me for the view of this long, very long needle that was to be inserted into my bone, just inside my top left buttock area.

Dr. Steinberg proceeded with sure movement and swift-ness, but I could tell that something seemed different to him. The first needle broke as it was being inserted. He hit the bone at an angle where it would not give, so he had to try again, then again. Twice breaking his needle and twice me thinking; "Oh my God … what is going on here?" The insertion part was painful for sure, but when he finally did achieve the right position, what was excruciating was the extraction process of my bone marrow itself. It is today still beyond my words to describe the pain. I was screaming, I mean **screaming** while this was being done. It took long seconds to finish, and I could tell it was most difficult for Dr. Steinberg as well. While it was happening I hid my face in the pillow, and I kept thinking to myself, *Stop screaming … stop screaming!* ***STOP IT!*** But I couldn't, it was by far the most painful, harrowing experience I have lived through to date. I am told that during my biopsy a woman coming down the hall to visit a loved one stopped as she heard me inside my room. She became extremely upset, crying out to the nurses, "**What are in the world are they doing to her in there?!**"

When it was over, I looked at Dr. Steinberg, who had sweat pouring down his face, and asked, "Did you get what you needed?"

He smiled, "I did, yes ... there is enough. I am so sorry for the pain you experienced, Stacey. It normally is not so painful, but given how high your white blood count is, I think this has contributed to the pain."

To soften with humor the fact that I had made such an unbelievable racket, I suggested to Dr. Steinberg that maybe this "little technique might be something the CIA should know about for interrogations."

Dr. Steinberg took a breath, smiled a sweet smile, under-standing I was trying to apologize. I blurted out then as I started rolling back around, "It's okay ... now that it is over, I don't feel anything, no pain at all!"

Loudly, Dr. Steinberg said, "Do not roll over yet, Stacey ... there is a lot of blood my nurse needs to take care of. In a few minutes when the anesthetic wears off, you will feel very sore, but it will be gone within a few days. And I need to forewarn you, we may need to do another one of these biopsies again soon."

I lay back down flat thinking, *Oh my, what is going to happen here?* It just started to hit me ... this "**thing**" was not going to be easy. Not easy at all!

Tom arrived a few minutes after I got cleaned up. He had driven down Rte. 95-S at eighty-five miles per hour. When he walked in the room, my heart just clutched. Smiling his wonderful smile with the twinkle in his eyes still there, but with a look of caution, my handsome, glorious husband sat down next to the bed on my right side and looked deep into my eyes. Tom asked softly, *"What is going on, beautiful?"*

I took a couple of deep breaths and reached for his hand, realizing in this moment that our life together was going to immediately change. I could feel my throat constricting and trying not to break down as I was forming the words … I said lightly, "I have leukemia."

Tom just stared at me for a long, long moment. Starting to feel tears for the first time I said, "I'm sorry, Tommy … I am so sorry; **I did not want to ever disappoint you like this.**"

Immediately Tom shushed me and grabbed at my hands, pulling on them. He bowed his head, tears coming very quickly. I will never forget not only Tom's first words, but how he looked at me when he said them. "It is okay, baby, I am here … **I am here!** You could not do anything to disappoint me. **We are in this together.**"

What I want to share in this book is my faith, my beliefs and the steps, and path that I had been on for long years prior to my diagnosis, which not only saved my life, but my mind and that of my family. Never in my life did I think I would ever suffer any kind of cancer, never mind leukemia. My family history is not one of cancers or any real serious illness at all. For about seven years during my thirties I was a vegetarian. My business was frozen seafood entrees, un-breaded and of exceptional high quality. I ate well, did therapeutic natural remedies like massage, chiropractic sessions, mud treatments for detox, I fasted, and I drank little to no alcohol and have never done recreational drugs in my life. I barely allowed myself an aspirin. So, how in the world did I get **LEUKEMIA?** Well, for sure my life in business was very stressful, and for sure I worked way too many hours, eighty hours each week. But, that part I felt was being offset by my other good strong daily habits. I went to bed early every night, and my home life with my family was peaceful. I thought I was bulletproof, without there being any chance, whatsoever, for me to develop a cancer or life-threatening illness. *But I did.* And it changed the trajectory of my life immediately and that of my husband's.

During the early days of my diagnosis, when it was determined that I had CML, Chronic Myeloid Leukemia, the treatment of choice for me was Gleevec, a smart drug known to be excellent in the targeting of leukemia, destroying only the cancer cells and allowing the good cells to live. Tom and I thought for a little while I was going to get off somewhat easy by way of this medication. Expensive, about $5,000 per month ... thank God for great insurance, which I had. As long as I kept up the medication I would live. But soon into the fight, my leukemia became aggressive, "blasting" as they call it, and my life took another sudden and unexpected turn.

Sitting in Dr. Steinberg's office one late October morning, about eighty days into my treatment with Gleevec, Tom and I noticed that Dr. Steinberg was not himself. Normally a very happy man, Dr. Steinberg was not smiling and he appeared pensive.

He explained, "Your leukemia has begun to blast, Stacey ... and we cannot get it under control. This is most serious, and I will need to transfer you to the care of Dr. Antin at Dana Farber."

Tom and I looked at each other, both knowing that Dana Farber is THE cancer hospital in New England. My thoughts went immediately to my memories of watching the Red Sox play and the incredible support and news regarding them and the Jimmy Fund. The Boston Red Sox are singularly one of the most outstanding contributors to this charity, of which Dana Farber is a recipient.

Dr. Steinberg began to speak again, snapping me back to the present. He added in a reassuring tone, "Dr. Antin is the Director of the Bone Marrow Stem Cell Transplant department there. He is an excellent doctor; you will be in good hands. You will need a stem cell transplant and you will need it very soon."

I asked why I could not have a transplant at Lahey and he explained that I needed an outside donor to "save my life" and that at Lahey the stem cell transplants were being done only from the patient's own stem cells, not those of a donor. "God willing," Dr. Steinberg added, "for you, there is one." He followed most solemnly, "This will change your life, Stacey. You will not be the same woman following this transplant. It will change your life. You need to prepare for that and be ready. Be brave, but be ready. When you meet with Dr. Antin, and I am arranging for that to happen as soon as his schedule allows, he will set the pace of this procedure and your only chance is to find a donor, hopefully one in your family."

Shell shock is how Tom and I felt and looked. We stared open mouthed at Dr. Steinberg, who was most sincerely disappointed for me. That was easy to see. I asked him several times if there was another option, and he said very sadly, "No."

I asked him, "How will this transplant change me?"

With a look of deep regret, he replied, "You are so vivacious, so full of life, Stacey. A transplant changes you. It affects your life's speed, what you can do, how you can do it. Some people never really recover; their immune systems stay very depressed. Their lives are saved, but they are changed. You will be changed." With that, he closed his file, wished me the very best, but told me I needed to go on to the next place being held for me at Dana Farber.

I could sense then just how it is with great doctors who develop affection for their patients, how painful it is when disappointments come along. I felt such respect for Dr. Steinberg and, at the same time, the beginnings of a deep sadness, a type which I had never felt before. Dr. Steinberg allowed Tom and me to remain in the room alone for a few minutes. We just sat there, staring off. Myself, I could feel a tangible "something" that I had never felt before growing inside me. I did not recognize its sensation at all. It was totally new and it felt dark.

"Grief," it was the early feelings of grief; I did not yet in that moment recognize it for what it was, but my inner body knew ... a type of death was coming and coming fast.

As Tom and I walked hand in hand, slowly and with some hesitant steps, back to the car, it was clear we both were deeply affected by Dr. Steinberg's words. Myself, I was becoming emotional. I was feeling fear for the first time since getting the diagnosis. Tom was gripping my hand hard. So hard, it was almost like he was sure, *just so sure* ... that in holding my hand, *that hard*, he could crush the leukemia right out of me. Together, as we continued walking, we knew our life was changing. Something close to panic began to come out in the air around us. But, seconds away, and when it was needed most, a "sign" was waiting. A sign that all would be well, that we were not alone, and that despite how scared we were both becoming, help, peace, and a trusting spirit were nearby, in fact ... right straight ahead.

As we approached my car parked with its trunk facing us, I gasped, "Oh MY ... TOM ... LOOK!"

Tom came up quick, his eyes having been focused straight down, and he jumped, as if I were about to fall or faint. He grabbed onto me, saying, "What is it! What?"

I said, "Look, look down!" When I pointed for him, Tom looked down at what I was seeing and there on the ground, right next to my car, facing the trunk, was a perfect large white feather.

"It's a White Feather, Tom!" I yelled. "Oh my God, do you know what this means?" Tom looked blank for a few seconds and stared at me like I was a little crazy, but then he slowly smiled, remembering vaguely that feathers hold a special spiritual meaning for me, and have for many years. It was my sign that God and my angels were near, and to not fear, no matter what. I picked up the feather, which was perfect, no dirt or rips in it. I looked around, but there were no other feathers anywhere, or by any other car, except this one in front of mine. It was Pure White. I could not tell what kind of bird it was from, but that did not matter; I brought it into the car and placed it between Tom and me. From that moment on, while there was much suffering still to come for us, I knew we were safe, and that I would come out of this okay. *Truly, I would be okay*. That however, did not stop the tears ...

I have come to learn that some people view illness as a punishment. Some view it as a curse from God or from Satan. Others don't know what to think, but they just know for certain that whoever has gotten sick probably deserved it for some reason or another. Judgment, doubt, fear, separation of the spirit, and separation between the family and the person who is ill, all can come into play, even by those in one's family who deeply love the person affected. Illness often arrives with a bang, and with a presence that calls everything in one's life to be put onto the table. Hiding, denial, tuning out, while this can happen for a little bit of time, cannot happen for long. Illness, when significant and prolonged, with recovery long and difficult, will yank everyone out of their locked closets, whether they want to come out or not. And the sunlight that hits everyone may not at first be welcome.

Secrets dissolve, inner character, good or bad, arrives for all to see, especially the patient, who sees for the most part *everything*. Very few people realize that even during the darkest hour after a prolonged coma, or severe drug inter-ference, a patient who is ill ... "sees" and they "see" things most people who have never been ill cannot imagine. They "see" truth. They see the truth that lies in their loved one's soul, regardless if it is pretty or ugly. They see the truth of their situation in the faces of their doctors and nurses, even before words get spoken. But with loved ones it just "IS" and it is appears without fail to *see* and be *seen*. And that can be the most beautiful thing and the most crushing to a patient. It was for me. Because often, those who you believe love you the most, or have known you the longest, cannot cope with the changes a disease like leukemia can bring.

For me, I could see in the faces of some who had known me the longest that seeing me so sick was not only painful ... but brought up for them their own fears for themselves. Faces would turn, eyes would look down, and shadows appeared. It was too much, it was too dif-ficult. And so I would lovingly let them walk away, and not ask them to be with me through this ... because inside, *I was never alone.* In the darkest hours of a long night in the hospital, after weeks of having been there, **I never felt alone**. Day after day, hour by hour, I had within me the spirit and the strength of a relationship I had built with God and my angels that sustained me, held me up, and kept me whole. And when I needed to feel their love and their touch the most, they were there. Through the many years of my life, since "they" first arrived, "HE" has always been with me.

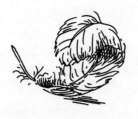

CHAPTER 2

The Beginnings: How I First Met God

I T WAS 1988, AND I WAS THIRTY YEARS OLD. I HAD BEEN BUILDING my company alongside my partner Andy since 1984. Together we had developed our manufacturing company as an offshoot of what had been two retail seafood stores. Andy had developed a unique seafood entrée/dinner that at the time was quite a new concept for the supermarket industry, and we were being asked by many retailers to sell our products to them. We met success at every turn, gaining approvals wherever we went; however, we had no idea how much money and capital starting a food company from scratch would take. So, we did everything. We catered, we delivered lobster bakes, we did shrimp cocktail delivery, and we ran two retail stores. We worked long hours, seven days a week, year after year, without a break. It was a very difficult time for us, but we were young and had a vital new product that screamed out for exposure, and so we ran behind this rush of constant evolving demand, trying desperately to keep up. While arduous, in the early days we had a lot of enjoyment and pleasure in the creative work we were doing together.

As time passed and things progressed, however, I became an insomniac. I probably lost two full years of sleep. Unable to slow my mind down at the end of a long day, I began a habit of falling asleep with the TV on, normally around 11:00 at night. I would sleep until around 1:00 AM and then with a start wake up and be fully awake. Thoughts on how to get through the next day would begin. At that time, we were personally $300K in debt. We had just moved a few years prior, in 1986, into an old Sealtest Ice Cream building in town, which had been built years earlier by Kraft Foods. While it was not a terrible expense monthly, we also had to purchase new equipment, and new packaging for our products. We needed to update, redesign, and rework over and over the products to fit the way the supermarket buyers wanted them to be merchandized. Constant demands were made for the company to find more and more money. Just when one hill was successfully climbed, Andy and I looked up to find another huge peak right smack in front of us.

It never ended – this cycle of building, climbing, and then seeing another incredible challenge. I was exhausted. Coping came often at night when I woke up at 1:00 AM on the dot every night. I would quiet my mind by writing a to-do list, scripting notes I needed to send to buyers, rewriting expenses needing to be paid, listing from memory the checks needing to be released and those released which needed to clear, and making lists of new customers to call. Usually, near 4:00 AM I would climb into bed and sleep until 6:30 AM, ready for work by 8:00 AM at the latest. Tired, I was bone-weary tired by the time I turned thirty. I can remember clearly on my thirtieth birthday driving to work in the morning, crying. I could not believe where I was in life. While I loved, loved, LOVED the work and the products Andy and I were developing, I just could not believe how heavy the burden was that I felt. I had never thought that at thirty years old I would feel like I was eighty, but I did. I would always gain energy though throughout the day because through it all, it is most exciting to have a new food item that buyers and consumers love. The letters we would receive revived me every day, and the words of encouragement from this retail chain, and that new retail chain, were incredible. So, I kept on. And I kept on. But the constant need to find more money in order to keep up with the high demands for new supplies, etc., just wore me down. Night after night, I could not sleep for more than a few hours. And the sleep that I did get was not deep enough. I could hear the TV in the background, but without it, I could not fall asleep at all. This unbreakable cycle continued for over two years.

Slowly, and without really noticing, I began to daydream about going to sleep and never waking up. Not sure how best to achieve that, I started to realize this seemed like a very good thing to figure out: finding a way to resolve my exhaustion by sleeping and never having to wake up again. I knew that I did not want to hurt myself physically; I just wanted to get unending sleep and the idea was becoming so intoxicating that it began to take on a life of its own. I would nearly swoon when I thought about how good such a deep sleep would be and to never wake up. THAT would solve all my stress and worries. I can recall clearly not really understanding at all what it was I was actually thinking. It was the effect, this feeling of longing that the daydream had on me that kept it alive. The sweet sensation and hope for "sleep." *I clung to it.*

As time passed, this daydream began to develop its own demands. And sure enough, I started to think about how best to make this desire for sleep, and to never wake up, happen. After months of this, I noticed that when I went to my car, there, right on the ground near my driver's side would be a small feather. I did not think anything of it, just got into the car and went. But after a while, I would see more of them, in front of my door at home, near the office door at the plant, and always every so often, right there next to my car door. I never picked any of them up, but I started to wonder where all these feathers were coming from.

The lack of sleep continued and the dream of going to sleep and never waking up became louder inside my head. Eventually, while at home I started to consider how best to achieve this goal. This yummy irresistible place ... where I did not need to wake up exhausted. To no longer have to deal with the constant issues of feeding a hungry growing company. *How to do it? How to get there?* And as things like this will develop, I began to plot it all out. I eventually decided I would just head to the local pharmacy and get as many sleeping pills as they had on the shelf. That should work, I felt. I would not actually injure myself, but I would finally have blessed sleep. So, I was firm and settled in my mind. I knew what to do and it felt to me like the right time. My plan began by me cleaning the house from top to bottom, placing new sheets onto my bed. (I have a sheet thing personally.) I love crisp, clean, newly washed sheets. So having new ones on the bed was a *must* for a good long sleep. I always slept the best when as a child my mom made my bed with clean new sheets. **Check!** I got that done, and then moved on to how best to take care of the rest of the house. While doing the dishes, I began to think through the final steps needed, which included my trip down the road to the pharmacy. I would do that last. A *click* happened for me in my head that was actually the final mental commitment lock. I was not daydreaming any longer; I was planning, and acting out my plan. I was not afraid at all; I was relieved. Soon ... I would be where I was craving. Peace and quiet, sleeping forever!

Just about at that exact moment, when I felt in my mind and heart that I was ready, I heard a man's voice speak to me. It was just over my left shoulder, and the words were actual words, sounds like anyone would make. Solid words; spoken out loud. The man said in a beautiful voice, *"Stacey, you are never alone, nor given any more than you can handle."*

I FROZE. I stopped moving completely, my breath caught in my throat, and the hairs on the nape of my neck stood straight up! My mind buzzed slightly as I slowly, very slowly turned to see what I knew beforehand was not there, *the man who just spoke to me.* There was no one there, nothing, but inside me I had an electrified sense that I was not alone there in my kitchen. I just breathed in and out, in and out, swallowing, trying to understand what had just happened.

What happened is that in a few short seconds, I was shaken out of my reverie. My whole idea of what I thought I was going to do vanished. Gone, it was gone. I woke up! I woke up from where I was and I was standing in my kitchen aware that I had just been awakened! By whom, I did not know. Shaking, I put down the dishcloth and slowly walked into my living room. Dazed but alert I tried to make sense of it. I can remember clearly that it only took about ten minutes for me to realize *I was going to have to face another day! Another day of no sleep, no rest, pure exhaustion!* And the burdens of running a company that needed so much more than I felt I had left to give. I became furious! Furious at this interruption in my plans that were so meticulously laid out and that I knew would have given me relief.

I fell to my living room floor and cried. I was crying so hard I began choking. The anger kept building too, and I was definitely afraid that I just might be going crazy. I begged this "voice," this whoever it was that so rudely interrupted me, to give me answers. "WHY? *Why did you come here like this?* WHY?" Over and over I asked the same question. After a bit of time when no other words were spoken to me, I just lay down on my floor and dissolved. I could not believe I was *not* going to be free, that I was *not* going to get out of this cycle of pain. I felt abandoned.

As I began to drift into a dreamlike state, I heard a different voice inside my head. Not the same as before, but pretty clearly I could hear the message that I was to go into my small den and to pick up a specific book that I had on the shelf. Too weak to disagree or think about where **this** message was actually coming from, I did go inside the den and retrieve the book. I found it within seconds. As I sat back down on my floor I opened the book and just fanned the pages. After a few times, I opened the book again and saw before me for the first time "St. Jude's Prayer." I read this prayer once and felt a light tingling sensation go through my body. The instructions were clear that this prayer should be read ten times when a miracle was needed. So I did that. I read the prayer ten times as follows:

O most holy apostle, St. Jude, faithful servant and

friend of Jesus, people honor and invoke you uni-
versally, as the patron of hopeless cases, of things
almost despaired of. Pray for me, for I am so hopeless and alone. Please help to bring me visible and
speedy assistance. Come to my assistance in this
great need that I may receive the consolation and
help of heaven in all my necessities, tribulations,
and sufferings, particularly (in my need for comfort and peace in this work that I am doing), and
that I may praise God with you always.

When I finished this prayer, I was calmer. I felt that
something had shifted inside my soul, my heart, and my
mind. In reading further down the page after the prayer I
saw that it was requested that you make a promise to St.
Jude, in return for the miracle being requested, a gift of
some kind in return. I immediately said out loud, "Dear
St. Jude, if you release me from this terrible pain that I feel,
and help me sleep and find the resources that I need to keep
the company going, I promise to feed and help any stray
animal that crosses my path. I promise!!" Silence followed
for several long minutes. And then once again I picked up
the book and scanned through it. Within a few minutes, I
came upon The Lord's' Prayer. I read the prayer, which I
knew by heart, a few times, speaking the words aloud.

Our Father who art in heaven, hallowed be thy
name. Thy kingdom come, Thy will be done, on
earth as it is in heaven. Give us this day our daily
bread. And forgive us our trespasses, as we forgive
those who have trespassed against us. And lead
us not into temptation, but deliver us from evil.

> For thine is the Kingdom, and the power and the
> glory, forever and ever. Amen.

The prayer and its words soothed me. So I kept reciting it over and over. In the following paragraphs, after the prayer, I read that The Lord's Prayer is the most powerful prayer ever given to mankind. That if it is said correctly, reverently, slowly, and with deep feeling, God would come without fail to be with you and to reside inside your soul and heart forever. I read The Lord's Prayer over and over countless times that night. Despair slowly turned into hope. Faint, but hope was there. I slept that night. It was a deep, restful sleep. I can remember the next day as I was preparing to go to work, asking myself, *Will a miracle be waiting for me today? Will the money that we need to get through the week just appear and be in our bank account?* Of course ... that did not happen, but what did happen soon after was certainly a miracle, a sign, and step by step, I grew to know God and his angels. I knew that for me personally, in order to keep this connection to God, I needed to pray with intent and feeling, and when I did, and I did it every day afterwards, my life and my problems slowly lessened.

You are wondering what miracles occurred? Well, I will tell you. There were many, so many, and I will share throughout this book a few of the most significant. Before I do, please know, and for certain many already do know, that prayer does not mean ... all problems simply disappear. What happens instead is that for the most part fear dissolves, exhaustion abates, and in tiny steps, the "choices" to you become clearer on how best to handle the trials that life places in everyone's path. The feeling of being all alone for me has been completely gone from my consciousness. That is by far, in and of itself, the greatest, most enduring gift. No one, no other human being has this ability to make me feel whole like this, nor does anyone have the power to take this peace and surety from me. No disappointment, and there were still many for me to experience, including leukemia, could rob me of this deep inner peace. In the years after meeting this angel in my home and finding God through prayer, small daily miracles have occurred, and even a few large startling ones, to remind me that when I did fall down (and we all do), God always, always was still with me.

Shortly following this time, within about six months, the first miracle of sorts did occur. Through a mutual friend in New York I met a gentleman who became a great friend and investor partner for me. On a handshake he gave me over $100K. This money proved very important as it enabled my small company to finally capture much better priced supplies. Inch by inch, step by step, daily I had in this gentleman a friend I could talk to, who had experience in business and who was always supportive, trusting, and dependable. I thrived under his friendship and his help, as did the company. Disappointments still came, and they came often, but I was handling them better, with more confidence and without fear. The food industry is gut-wrenchingly difficult. The statistics for success are just awful. In the first year of trying to get new food items onto the supermarket shelves, 92% of startups fail. Those that do survive, within five years, at least 50% fail. The fact that we had so many interested retailers did not blunt or stop this difficulty. Growth means constant new monies and resources are needed. It is 24/7, and the demands never end. While I prayed daily, I still suffered from being overtired; as the workload for me was intense. My mind always was thinking, planning, re-planning, etc. I hung in, but it wore me down.

One day, as I was once again driving in Massachusetts to visit my Purity Supreme buyer, I realized I was way too exhausted and feeling low again. It was mid-morning when I arrived at their offices and learned, after waiting for over an hour, that the buyer was delayed for about four hours. "Would you please come back later this afternoon?" the receptionist asked. I was deeply disappointed, as I had to be back into the office later to handle several important items, but I accepted and indicated I would be back at 3:00 PM, and then went out to my car.

Once there, I lay back my head and just wilted. I was very tired and in general dispirited by my heavy workload and responsibilities. This delay today was not going to help things at all. It was about a year after the visit with my angel at home, and while I was strengthened by prayer, I still had to work very hard every day, and it was a most tiring kind of work. This was before anyone had cell phones by their side, email, or iPads, never mind GPS in the car or on the phone as an application. Instead of it taking one hour to do a dozen tasks, I needed three or four hours. It is easy to forget today, with all of the convenient tools we have to help us, how long simple tasks took back in the late 1980s and even early 1990s. We had fax machines, but they used thermal paper and often they had issues. Overnight mail was available but it was very expensive. Our PCs were slow and often had to be serviced. There simply were none of the internet connections between businesses or websites that enhance every office today. Often tasks required several hours before they could be completed.

Knowing that I would be working again very late that

night, I turned on the car to listen to the radio and then decided to pull out of the parking lot, to head off and find something to eat. Normally, I would have shot back up onto the highway to look around for a restaurant right off one of the exits, but instead I took one of the side roads and just drove. Sort of not fully alert, nor thinking about anything specific, I can recall seeing after several miles this very small, almost tiny (doll-like) white house sitting on the lawn in front of what looked to be a bigger house behind it. I pulled over because the sign read "Subs." I got out and walked up the small pathway to the tiny door and I remember thinking, *is this possible? Did someone build this little house in front of their house to open a sub shop?* Inside, the ceiling was very low and the walls short. There really was only enough room for me to stand alone, with the counter facing me. The man I saw with his back to me had snow white hair, he was tall, a little bulky, but when he turned around, I gasped. He had the palest white skin and the brightest blue eyes I had ever seen. He said not a word, just nodded to me to see what I wanted. I ordered a turkey sub with lettuce and when he turned back to get my sandwich ready, I can remember feeling again that same sensation I had in my kitchen. It was a feeling of light electricity going through my body. I noticed how incredibly tiny the walls were, and when I turned to my right, I saw a poster that in a normal house would not be so large looking, but this poster covered the wall almost entirely. It was a picture of a beach with only two footprints in the sand. As I started to focus, I saw there was writing, a prayer-type poem I began to read. Within seconds, tears began to run down my face. I was silent, I did not cry out, but I was so deeply affected

I felt my body starting to hum. Tears almost blinding me poured down ...

The prayer describes a soul upon death walking along a beach with the Lord and seeing scenes from his/her life just lived. On the sand for many miles there were two sets of footprints in the sand, but during those desperate times when life was so hard, there was only one set of footprints to be seen. The soul cried out to the Lord asking WHY during those most terrible and lonely times did the Lord abandon the soul, leaving him/her to walk alone. The Lord gently replied that he would never have left and that during those times when only one set of footprints was on the sand, he, the Lord, had been carrying the soul.

I do not remember anything distinct after that, except that I came to myself, in the car, with a finished sandwich in my lap. The feeling I had inside me was full-blown warmth and incredible deep love. As I started to become more alert I realized I was driving down the rest of this long road I had been on. Curious about what had occurred to me, I decided I needed to go back and see this small sub shop again. I had plenty more time before my appointment, so I turned around and while thinking about the prayer and the wonderful feelings of incredible love exploding in my heart, I sensed intuitively that this delicious afterglow was like maybe having been near to God. While I was reading the prayer, I felt inside me that *God was speaking those words directly to me!* The words had felt alive!

I had to find this tiny house again.

After driving up and down the street, I could not relocate this small house or the sign that said "Subs." Up and down the street I drove, slowly, looking closely at every house for anything familiar. I saw nothing. I thought for a minute I recognized the pathway and the house that sat behind, but no ... the tiny white house was just not there. It was not anywhere on the street. I became a little worried as I was searching because I realized just then that I could not recall at all how I had paid for my sandwich. "Did I??" I was not certain. I had no memory of having done so, or of having eaten the sandwich. So, I headed back to Purity Supreme's parking lot where I could think about what had happened. For several hours I sat in a quiet area of the parking lot and reflected. I went over the entire experience again and again. The intense feeling of warm, calm love was still with me and when I focused on that sensation, I knew I would never find a logical explanation. What I did sense for absolute certain is that I had been kissed by heaven in a way that would stay with me. I felt a deep inner peace that could not be denied and I was feeling totally refreshed. The expression "God works in mysterious ways" kept ringing in my head; my grandmother would say that so often when I was younger. But, more importantly, I felt "touched," and this feeling had sunk deep inside me.

On this day, I feel I was again "saved." Saved in the truest sense of the word, but there is more, much more for me that has been miraculous.

My life in business continued. I traveled, we opened more supermarkets to our products, and in general, daily events attained a rhythm all around that stabilized my life. Financial difficulties had eased tremendously and I began to have in my life the resources I needed not only for the business, but for myself so that I could relax and enjoy the fruits of my labors. Personally, I did not date a lot after a long-standing relationship ended in the mid-'90s. I simply did not have a lot of spare time and I found myself unwilling to be involved in casual relationships. A lot of men that I met really did not know what to make of me. Often I would be on a date and the conversation was more like an interrogation. "How many employees do you have? How much do you book a year in sales? How do you open up new accounts? What kind of profits do you make? How much do you collect a year in salary?" and on and on it would go. Sometimes these rapid-fire questions were asked of me before dinner was even ordered! I can remember on one of these dates making a decision that lasted for almost seven years ... to not date again, unless I met the man I really wanted to be with. This decision happened when after the fourth attempt at dating, the gentleman I was with could not slow down his questions and he appeared almost not interested in me at all, only my business. I got up from the table shortly after we sat down and apologized, saying to him directly, "I do not want to do this tonight. I am leaving now; please do not call me again." Staring at me with shock, he tried to apologize, but I could not continue in his company. I was fed up with wasting my time on men more fascinated with my business than with me. And I am very glad I did do this, because in the years following, I grew closer and closer to God. And when I was ready ... I met Tom, the absolute love of my life.

I spent almost every weekend between the ages of thirty-six and forty-two resting, reading, and visiting my mom. I have in my life a handful of very close friends that I cherish. I would travel a lot for the business, spending when I could a long weekend somewhere beautiful. This worked great for me. And of course, many stray and injured animals always did come across my path. Holding true to my promise years prior to St. Jude, I had throughout these years rescued dozens of cats, dogs, and other small wildlife. I had two great veterinarians near where I lived, and as needed, which was with some regularity, they helped me with the animals that I found or that came to my door. Many times when trying to find a good home for one of the animals, I went to our local SPCA, in Stratham, New Hampshire, which is a wonderful place. These experiences with rescues enriched my life deeply and helped bring balance into my soul.

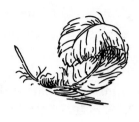

CHAPTER 3

The Struggle to Understand the "Why" of My Illness

S O MUCH OF MY LIFE, AND THE DAILY LIVING OUT OF MY FAITH through good works and being true to myself, prepared me in the years leading up to 2009 to endure the difficult challenge that is leukemia. The medical miracles today that are being performed for patients who have leukemia, who only a decade or two earlier would have died, enthrall me. But despite how good my chances could be with a stem cell donor, several weeks passed during November 2009 before Tom and I knew for sure if I had one. And during these weeks Tom and I went through hell.

We spent hours together talking about what was to come for us. To be with me through this whole time, Tom had taken an extended leave of absence at work, both from US Airways and FlightSafety. It was incredibly strengthening for me to have Tom by my side during doctors' visits and to just be next to me almost every minute of each day. His constant presence enabled me to experience him as my husband in a way I had not really ever fully captured before. *My husband* ... it took on a new meaning for me. I came to understand, deep in my heart, what that word truly meant ... *husband*. Wow, what a gift.

But as the hours passed during each day, traumatic emotions about my upcoming transplant would appear quite suddenly for Tom. While Tom knew I believed all would be well, and that I would live, he was afraid. He was deeply afraid and he was at times very angry. He could not understand "why" our incredible life together was to be sidelined by this horrible disease, with a YEAR of recovery minimum. In fact, the truth is we both knew from what we had been told to expect that setbacks during the first year would occur, and in actuality a patient does not really begin to be fully well until after year three of recovery. A long time!

Knowing this, Tom asked me constantly "why" this had happened. Being raised Catholic; Tom readily admitted to me early in our relationship that he struggled with feelings of guilt. Guilt for what ... he could never really say, but always a little bit of guilt seemed just around the corner in his life. In general, this never really came up for us in any harmful way, but there it was though, in the little things that were just Tom. For example, if we were going to have a really great dinner, Tom wanted first to do something physical or something that would make him sweat or get him dirty, like working out in the garage on his car or his boat or in the building of something useful. Tom likes contrasts. If he is to enjoy a nice dinner and a bottle of wine, then beforehand he has to feels he's "earned" it, by doing something laborious. This never reached a level of intensity that disturbed me, but it was just funny how he was. It was a constant in our life together. So, in trying to make sense of how this awful disease came to be inside of me, Tom searched for answers. And his first inclination was to feel that maybe, just maybe for some strange reason, it was retribution for something he had done or I had done. And in Tom's search for answers we spent hours together revisiting our personal lives before we met and our life together, which by then had lasted seven years.

Our marriage from the start had been a very happy one. We traveled everywhere in the first three years together, staying at wonderful resorts; we went to Paris and London a few times, Bermuda, California, Florida, Guam, etc., and just had together everything we needed. While we enjoyed friends, we did not need to have a lot of them around. Tom and I love being together, alone and with each other. Our daily habits are similar. We are immensely compatible. Truly we are best friends and mates in the deepest sense of the word. I often think that meeting each other later in life was for us a good thing, even though this can sometimes mean a lot of baggage bleeding into the new relationship. We decided early on to deal with that by not allowing either of our respective pasts to interfere in our future together. We each had experiences in our lives that contributed to who we were now as adults, and neither of us could reset the hands of time, transporting us back to a new reset point (no matter how much we wished it were possible). We agreed that we would leave our pasts at our new front door, with the big exception being Tom's two children, Christina and Jeffrey. They were with us in every way right from the beginning.

So we started anew. And it worked. Tom and I let nothing that was not a part of our life together affect us, and consequently we felt lighter and less trapped by things that were over and done with forever.

This reality, which became for Tom and me our life together, meant we knew each other very well. We could finish each other's sentences; we "felt" what each other wanted and needed beforehand. In fact Tom had an interesting ability to know just how I was doing every day when he came home from work just by holding me and smelling my skin and hair. Instantly, he could detect if I was feeling down or upbeat or whether I felt tired. Almost always, he was correct. Most of our daily life was fluid and easy, and almost always I felt very good. But Tom knew when I was not feeling so great, and I think this ability of his held a deeper answer as to how my becoming sick with cancer affected him so profoundly, much more so than what his outer appearance would indicate. In reality, Tom was deeply traumatized. So watching Tom struggle for answers on the "why" of it all was difficult. We spent days in a circular discussion about it, with me wanting so much for Tom to have a sense of peace and to trust. We spoke often on the question of "why cancer," but we did not really get anywhere. Then one day over coffee, Tom addressed me with a distinct question. **"Are you being punished?"** he asked with a direct look as if *I certainly had to know this answer*. I replied gently, "No, of course I am not being punished. Why would you think that?"

Tom said, "I don't know; I just cannot stop thinking that this disease, which is so awful, should not have happened to a person like **you**!!! **It's not FAIR!!**" He was crying, totally convinced something "bad" had to have been done for this to have arrived in our life.

I trusted then the words that came to me. "Is it

possible ... at all possible, Tom ... if we believe in the goodness of God, that this may all be happening for **your** benefit? Could it be for you, Tom? If we believe that illness comes as a teacher, (and I do), then maybe, the lesson is not only for me ... but *for you as well?* Maybe, there is *'something'* *God has in mind for you specifically* and I am the facilitator of this lesson, *meant for you*, because we love each other so much?" Tom stared at me with stunned amazement when I said that, saying absolutely nothing in return. We had been sitting in our living room that morning and Tom sat back then on the couch and sighed deeply, closing his eyes.

My beautiful husband is a kind and generous man, but throughout his life, he had few difficult struggles. He wanted to become a pilot since he was eight years old, and so he did: flying for the Air Force as a bomber and tanker pilot and then heading off to become an airline for US Air. My husband so enjoys flying, and his work, that I have often said that when he comes home from a long trip, he looks ten years younger. He is *that* happy in what he does. It is infectious really. His love of flying inspires me. To be with someone who really loves what they do for work is a joy. But living like this for the most part does shelter one from the understanding that comes when you have struggled or been through tremendous pain, the kind of pain that softens the soul and makes one truly empathetic.

As Tom sat with his eyes closed, the living room was deeply quiet. With the sounds of our wooden clock ticking in the background, and the beautiful morning light coming in through our windows, I asked Tom to consider how "blessed his whole life had been. That maybe; God wanted for him to *feel things deeper*, be more *sympathetic and understanding of the troubles others have*. And maybe this journey that we would walk together was really meant for him? Possibly in the walking of it, Tom would learn and grow?" I can remember how still Tom became. He thought on this a long time. I could see that he knew I was sincere in my words. He also knew that I was not afraid to die and he knew the reasons why, which I am going to share and are part of the motivation to write my story. But before I do that, know that Tom was at a precipice. He had to make a choice. He had to either accept or believe that only good would come of my illness and my recovery, or he would sink like a stone into despair. He had to make the decision himself. And for a man used to life flowing easily like a perfect sheet of music, this was beyond words difficult.

True to myself, I spoke bluntly and in honest terms. "I could die, Tom, I might die and you know that I am not afraid to die. Knowing that about me, I do not want to see you, no longer able to live without me. You must *choose* to trust in order to remain strong or your fear will demoralize you, and I need for you to remain strong – to stay strong with me. This road will not be easy, but I need for you to try."

This did not immediately help Tom, who was terrified that *I would die!* He made it clear to me that he did not want to be left alone on Earth without me. He was losing hope. He was moving steadily towards a total emotional breakdown.

As I watched Tom's face and the changing landscape his fear was creating, I was suddenly pulled back into my own memories, on how I had felt, just a few months earlier, when sudden and abrupt fear arose in me that Tom had possibly died in a plane crash.

It was January 15, 2009, around 3:40 in the afternoon. I was working on my emails at the kitchen table when my older brother Billy sent an email message to me. "**Sis, is**

Tom flying today? A US Airways plane just crash landed into the Hudson River." With shock, I re-read Billy's email. Tom WAS FLYING and was actually, at about this exact time, due to land in New York at LaGuardia Airport! I can recall vividly the feeling of my complete lower body, into my legs, melting totally. The sensation was like hot liquid. If I had been standing I would have fallen. I replied back, "YES, and he is supposed to be landing in NY just about **now!**" Billy sent back, **"get the TV turned on!!!"**

I made it to the living room on very shaky legs, turned on the TV, and there on the screen was a US Airways Airbus 320, Flight 1549, bobbing in the cold water. I could not breathe at all. I had throat-gripping fear. I had an awful feeling that this was Tom's plane. All I knew was he was scheduled out of Boston that day on the 3:00 PM shuttle to LaGuardia. I did not have his flight number, which sometimes he did leave for me. This was a routine type of flight so there did not seem to be any need. I continued watching the news and as of yet, on my station, there was no information as to the reasons for the crash or what happened to the crew and passengers. For long minutes it seemed, as I waited to see something more, my mind (heaven help me) kept putting images up of a car driving into the yard in front of our house, with uniformed men and a priest coming to tell me Tom had died. I imagined being at his funeral, of all our families and friends, and the awful days and months following of being without him. I was devastated, living a nightmare I never thought I would ever see happening to us. It was a profound sense of doom. It was then that I picked up the phone and called my mom. My hands were shaking so badly, I could not dial very well and had to start over three times. Mom finally was there and when she heard me, she said immediately, "it is okay, Stacey, everyone has gotten out."

I screamed, "Why is my station not reporting that?" At about this moment a banner came up on the screen with phone numbers for US Airways families to call for information, and another for people who had relatives on the plane as passengers. I saw the flight number as 1549, but I did not know whether it was Tom's. Mom calmed me and within a few minutes, I was able to dial the US Airways number being flashed. I was surprised when the call was answered immediately. I blurted out, "My husband is a pilot for US Airways and he was on a shuttle flight into LaGuardia that left Boston at 3:00 PM. I don't know his flight number." She requested his name. In seconds she said "No, Flight 1549 is not his plane." The relief I felt was immediate. I sat down on my couch and put my head into my hands. It was pounding. I felt drunk. I almost vomited. As I went into the kitchen to get a drink of water, I realized that I had totally freaked out and I began to feel a sense of shame at having traveled so far off into my mind imagining that Tom was dead and seeing his funeral in my mind. I felt I had no self-control and that I had behaved like a drama queen ... something I loathe.

Tom was still in the air at this exact time, circling over LaGuardia. All planes in the air near LaGuardia had been put into a holding pattern, and all flights due to take off were "held" on the ground. I tried to contact Tom, not knowing any of this, but his cell was not turned on. I left three messages for him to call me when he could. As it happened, Tom's crew was not told anything about the crash, only that they were to divert back to Boston. When Tom landed on the ground in Boston, and during their taxi back to the gate, he called me. I told him what I knew from the news. All he said that he and his crew knew was the information streaming over their internal communication messaging in the cockpit, that a "US Airways plane had crashed into the Hudson." No reason was indicated as to why. Tom needed to say goodbye to me as soon as he knew I was calmer, as he and his crew were being instructed to reposition for a new departure time that would be set soon.

My mind left the memory of that cold January day, and settling back on my living room couch with Tom, I decided to keep myself quiet. Watching Tom, who was still within his own thoughts, *I understood!* Seeing him suffer with a dread that I might die … I fully understood. I remembered well just then how I had felt for that short, but horrible, hour. And for the first time, I was thankful for having had that experience. I had a better grip on what I was witnessing. Tom's agony was much worse, though, than what I had gone through, because the not knowing for him regarding what might actually happen to me had been escalating now for weeks. It was snowballing inside him and he was suffocating.

After long minutes had passed, I moved forward and put my arms around Tom and held him. It was clearer to me that I could not make any of the visions he was prob-ably playing and replaying inside his head stop, but I had the hope they would ease. I kept thinking that if we treated this whole thing going forward like a "military operation" and did not dwell on whether I might die, we would pull through this. To help Tom best, I did not try to go where he was in his mind. I needed to not do that. I could not swallow his horrible fear and pain into me, because if I did, I too would begin to drown, and thankfully, I knew better than to do that. Drowning in the fear was not the answer.

Rising above it was. In an attempt to do that, I just kept talking with Tom about the exceptional spiritual experiences that I had been through, throughout my life, which had locked me into this place of calm that Tom could *see*, but did not feel himself, and ... he was desperate for it.

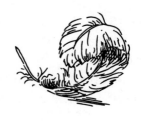

CHAPTER 4

The Divine Experience That Changed My Life Forever

N 2001, DURING A BUSINESS TRIP IN NAPLES, FLORIDA, SHORTLY before I met Tom, I suffered a pulmonary hemorrhage. There was no real medical conclusion reached while I was in the hospital those three weeks regarding what exactly caused this hemorrhage to occur. Some years later, there was a potential connection made concerning my having been injured due to exposure to very high levels of ozone from defective purifiers that had been in my home. And while physically it would have been good to have known the reasons why this event happened, emotionally it was no longer relevant to me because through this experience, I came out the other side of the long difficult path that had been my life up until then.

It began in late April 2001. I left Manchester, New Hampshire, in the early morning and headed off to Tampa,

Florida, for a meeting later that week with Publix Supermarkets. I visited with my good friend Kathy, who also worked for my company in retail sales. We have a deep connection, Kathy and I. Kathy herself had struggled with health issues during this time and was in many ways on the same spiritual path as I was. We read a lot of the same inspirational books; we prayed together and believed many of the same things. Our goal as friends was to keep on keeping on, helping each other stay on the path. Living as authentic and true as we could, our goal was to live out our spiritual beliefs every day, by the small things that were genuine and based in truth, even if it was as simple an act as just feeding a stray cat. By being a positive light in our own lives and in the lives of others, Kathy and I, while we were not perfect, knew if we remained committed to certain spiritual truths we would reduce the suffering we had been experiencing in life to date. Suffering just "is" part and parcel of why we are here on this earth, we believed. Without suffering a soul does not grow, and Kathy and I together helped each other grow. We leaned on each other and read a lot of the same books, like those by Marianne Williamson, White Eagle, and Lynn Andrews.

After a few days in Tampa, my schedule was to head down into Naples to visit other business associates early in the week, and then drive back into the Lakeland area mid-week. For the weekend, I had made plans to spend a couple of nights at a nice hotel right on the water in Naples. It was beautiful weather that week and I had begun my first day by taking a really nice long hike along the walking bridge that connected the hotel to the beach. It ran along well-developed vegetation, flowers, bird sanctuaries, and small streams of water. I swam and had a truly relaxing afternoon under the beach umbrella, reading and snoozing.

It was so peaceful, the water was luscious, the fruit drinks were incredibly refreshing, and the views beautiful. The sky was that robin's egg blue with small white puffy clouds that makes Florida so special. I had a wonderful first day.

Around 4:00 PM I headed back to my room to shower and give thought as to where to have dinner. I did not know if I wanted to head out and grab something light or to just hang in and watch a movie. At around 5:30 PM, I ended up making the decision to order room service, pick out a movie, and chill. On the balcony while overlooking the red and terracotta rooftops all around me, I ordered onion soup, salad, and an iced tea. When dinner came I asked the waiter to set it up on the table outside on the balcony. It was perfect weather and I was very relaxed. About halfway through my dinner, though, I lost my appetite and pushed my food away. Standing back up, I noticed that my vision was not as good as it was a few moments earlier. The rooftops that I had been so enjoying seemed not quite so distinct. Hazy, it was as if a veil was now over my eyes. I was puzzled. I could not really understand why I felt this sudden change in my vision, which interfered with what had been a very cozy feeling of contentment.

I went back into my room and decided to lie down on the couch. It seemed a little early to start a movie, so I picked up a magazine to flip through. More trouble continued with my vision. The pages seemed to move and I was having a hard time focusing. I looked up at the walls and the pictures seemed okay, not too fuzzy. I began to think maybe I had gotten too much sun earlier. A huge fan of long baths, I decided then that I needed one. After another hour passed, I noticed that I was not yet getting back to myself and so I climbed into my beautiful bed. The sheets were wonderful, cool and crisp. I snuggled in and decided to just get some sleep. While starting to drift off, I had the idea to put a pillow under my upper back. I thought maybe it would not be comfortable, and almost decided not to do it, but I tried it and it was most comfortable. I fell asleep quickly and slept soundly until around 6:00 AM.

When I got up to head off to the bathroom, I noticed in the mirror that I looked absolutely awful. My face was puffy and I appeared a bit gray in color. Within seconds, I coughed and spittle of blood came up, bright red into the sink. I was stunned. Almost immediately, another cough and this time I put my hands together, catching a good amount of hot red blood. I looked up into the mirror and was stunned to see that I had blood now on my chin and neck. A cycle began of me coughing up more blood to the point where for a second, as I was trying to catch my breath, I would immediately cough up more blood. I realized if I was not careful, I might inhale my own blood by breathing in at the wrong moment. Remembering when I was younger and a swimmer, I knew I could hold my breath for a long time and be okay. I immediately held my breath until after I coughed up blood, and then breathed in. The cough-ups continued.

I picked up the phone and called the front desk telling them that I was in distress, coughing up blood constantly, and that I felt I needed an ambulance. They said someone would be up to the room immediately. I headed off to the closet to get dressed. While in front of the mirror I coughed again, and blood fell onto the white carpet. It is funny what the mind thinks while in a crisis, but my first thought was *that will cost me, no way is the hotel not going to charge me for a blood stain that probably will not come out.* My second thought was to get dressed as fast as possible for fear I might pass out and the hotel staff would find me half dressed in a pool of my own blood on their beautiful white carpet.

Almost immediately there was a knock at the door and the gentleman who had come up called immediately on his phone verifying my condition. He indicated into the phone that "a white woman, around the age of forty" was definitely coughing up blood. Dressed now and ready to go, I can remember saying to myself, *Boy, I really must look terrible for him to say I appear around the age of forty!* For the most part, people always thought I was a good seven years younger than I actually was. No thought inside my head yet as to "why" I was coughing up so much blood. It was not until I was in the ambulance that I started to consider this question.

The firemen and the ambulance guys were fantastic to me. Once I was settled, the paramedic in the back said to the driver, "Head to Cleveland instead," and I asked with alarm, "You're taking me to Cleveland, Ohio?" And he laughed, saying, "No, no ... there is a brand new hospital called The Cleveland Clinic, and we are taking you there instead."

Within minutes of arriving at this new hospital I was transported into the ER. The hospital was beautiful, quiet, with no other patients around that I could see. A doctor came in to examine me, but for several hours no one knew exactly what to make of the blood or its cause. The plan was to watch me longer. I continued to cough up blood, but it seemed less than before. So I was transferred into another examining room with another doctor. Several more hours passed. While they were a very nice group of hospital staff, the feeling with them seemed a bit disconnected. As though not one of them knew what to make of my condition and after a little while, I heard them discussing releasing me. I was panic stricken. How could they even consider such a thing, and I requested that they wait. Within an hour the cycle of coughing up more blood began again with more intensity and immediately I was admitted into a private hospital room. I learned a bit later that since the hospital had only been open for one week, the pulmonary team was not yet there at the time that I was admitted. So, the hospital staff, while concerned for me, did not really know what to do next. Until they did they felt it best to handle me as if I had an exotic virus or bacterial infection, and so I was admitted into an isolated room.

By far, this was the most beautiful hospital room I had ever seen. The walls were a gorgeous soft green and on the walls there were colorful pictures, and the bathroom had an incredible marble-looking finish. The towels were plush and most importantly the bed had pretty good sheets. I was made to feel comfortable. I was confused, but comfortable. I had no idea what was going on with me. About thirty minutes after getting into my room, I met a hospital staff doctor who examined me. I kept trying to explain to her that I had a funny sensation behind my back when blood would come up, but she continued to focus her examination on my throat area, chest area, etc. They did blood work and took a chest x-ray. The nurses and the doctor began to wear masks. Throughout the day, there were no answers and for the most part I was left alone. By early afternoon, I had put a call into Kathy and asked her to help me with my hotel room and my rental car. She came down into Naples immediately to help settle things with both. At the same time, out of an abundance of caution, she contacted my buyer at Publix and indicated I would need to postpone my meeting. In all the years of doing business with this wonderful account, I had never been late or cancelled an appointment. The buyer sensed something was not right, and asked Kathy repeatedly what was going on with me. Kathy was appropriately discreet, saying nothing about my having been admitted into the hospital, but she did tell him she would keep him posted as he requested she do.

Throughout the day I felt frustration with the doctors, who seemed to have no clue what was going on with me. Kathy came by the hospital room later in the afternoon to see me. She sat with me for several hours and together we tried to figure out what my condition was. I ordered dinner, but I did not have any appetite. I can remember how comforting it was to have Kathy with me. She, like me, was not easily provoked into panic, and with her easy manner and sweet nature, I remained calm. I looked at the wall clock, it was 5:00 PM, and I was getting very, very tired. I had been coughing up a constant flow of blood all throughout the day and it was wearing me out. The nurses had given me earlier a small bucket to cough into and it by now was just not large enough, so they brought into my room a large plastic trash container, similar to one I had in my kitchen at home. The nurse told me casually to "just lean over and cough into that." I was a little amazed by her demeanor, but what other choice did I have? One hour passed, and then another and I continued to cough up blood.

By 7:30 PM I was getting too tired to continue my visit with Kathy, and so I asked if she wouldn't mind leaving so I could rest. The plan was for her to stay in my hotel room that night, pack my things, and get them over to me in the morning. After Kathy left, I began to watch the wall clock, which was right in front of me, slightly to the right. More time passed and still no slowdown in what I realized now was a severe hemorrhage. I was quickly filling up the trash container. My vision was progressively getting worse and I started to feel like I was losing my grip on reality. The nurses and hospital staff had left me alone during this entire period of time. It was quiet in my room, very quiet. By 9:00 PM I was aware that I was not breathing very deeply. I was breathing shallowly, unable to take deep breaths and a feeling like being drunk began to overcome me. "Something is definitely wrong," I said to myself; I felt like I was fading ...

Time continued to pass when suddenly ... *"something"* arrived. A sudden charge happened in the air of my room. A feeling came over me. I could sense a "presence," a "shadowy" type feeling right behind me. It had a strong presence, a dark presence even, not evil, but dark in that it was profoundly strong. Many times amplified, as is the feeling you sometimes have when you know someone is standing right behind you. This is what I felt. I knew within a few short seconds that this presence was "death" and that it had come for me. My body, which was exhausted by now, started to feel fear and I involuntarily curled into the fetal position. My thoughts were clear: *I am not going to make it to the morning. I am going to die. I am forty-two years old and I am going to die. What a shame,* I said to myself. My body began to feel more fearful, and I thought to myself, *I don't want to feel pain.* My mind seemed to be working as it normally did, and the voice inside me was still the same as always. I can remember saying to myself, *now I know why "death" is portrayed in* A Christmas Carol *as a dark shadow because death's presence is so strong, its power feels dark.* But I knew it was good; I could sense that very clearly.

Then, as the minutes slowly slipped by, I felt a gentle, *an ever so elegant touch*, the lightest of touches ... this "presence" moved from the tip of my head slowly down the entire right side of my body. It felt like the flowing of water, all the way down, gentle ... ever so gentle was this touch, until it reached the end of my feet. When completed, I unfolded and lay back flat onto the bed. I was able to take a deep full breath. A glorious breath! Like nothing in my life I had ever been able to do for myself, this breath was so complete, so delicious a feeling, I was ecstatic inside. My eyes were closed and I was reveling in this feeling. When I opened my eyes the only thing I could see was that all around me was a white cloud. Only pure white was what I saw, like being inside a cotton ball. I closed my eyes again and reopened them a few seconds later. I saw the wall clock quite clearly, but the angle seemed a bit different than what I had remembered from earlier. It looked lower to me. I closed my eyes again, feeling a wonderful sense of delicious peace.

When I opened my eyes again, there at the foot of my bed stood a man. I could see him very distinctly. He wore a long white cotton coat. He had on glasses and was holding a clipboard in his hands. He said not a word. He did not smile at me; he did not move ... he was just *there*. I stared at him for what seemed a long time, while still feeling this wonderful sense of relief and comfort. I had stopped coughing up blood and was still deep inside myself and my own mind. I realized slowly then that this man was an angel. After this realization hit me, my first thought was *why is he not shining? I thought angels were supposed to shine?* Gently we looked at each other and while looking, I focused on the clipboard he was holding and instantly knew that my life, all of it as I had lived it, was there in his hands.

Without moving his lips, he began to speak to me. *Stacey, you have done well.* As he said these words I saw on the left side of the wall the outline of a door being formed by a whirl of swirling colors. It was indistinct and hazy, but the outline was clearly becoming that of a door. The angel continued to speak directly into my mind: *You have done well, and you are being given a choice. You may stay ... or you may come home.*

I did not answer immediately or attempt to speak; I just kept looking at him ... *wondering*. He remained still. He did not move, he did not smile, and he in no way did anything to affect the *choice* that he said I had. I saw then that he was a most loving, beautiful spirit ... gentle beyond words. I looked back at the door, which was beginning to change colors, becoming much clearer. I could feel a pull ... a part of my soul longed to "go home" ... and **he** knew that. I knew he knew that I longed for the peace going **HOME** would bring. There was no feeling of time, or of the need to rush. Peacefulness, contentment, wholeness is all that I felt.

In truth, I did not know whether I wanted to stay in this life or not. I began to think about how difficult my life had been, of the business controversies I was drowning in with my partners whose strong disagreements could not, it seemed, be healed.

I asked through my mind, "Why have I suffered so? WHY??" The angel did not answer. There was silence. For long moments, he just looked at me, not moving or saying more. I thought about the repetitive issues and recent days again of difficulty and I knew **HE** knew all of this, and allowed me to revisit them in my mind. When I asked **WHY** again, he said to me, *there is perfection in either choice. You may stay or you may come home.* He gave me then a vision whereby I could see my family, my mom and my brothers, as they would be following my death. They would be okay, that I could see! I knew that they all would be okay and he was showing me that I did not need to worry. He then said very clearly, *you are not to stay for them! Know that all will be well.* I thought immediately that I did not want to feel any pain in the act of dying. The angel heard these thoughts and said ... *you will feel no pain.*

I knew instantly in that moment that all I needed to do if I decided to leave was reach my arm for the door and I would be gone. I would leave my body fully and I would enter heaven. On the other side I could feel beauty and peace awaited me. I could sense that clearly. I did not know yet, though, what I wanted to do. I just knew I wanted the pain that had been a long part of my life to end, and in that moment, the face of one of my business partners appeared before me, a man with whom I was having such terrible struggles. It seemed his role in my life was constantly that of the antagonist. Or so I thought. His face, which was right in front of me, clear and true, was smiling at me. A wonderful beaming smile filled with total love was pouring out of him. I looked at my angel and I said to him from my mind, *what is this bastard doing here?? Why is he here, now, at this private moment for me?* I was angry and confused by his intrusion. A moment passed and my angel then gently extended his hand. When he opened his palm, I could see a ball of string, tied into a knot. He said lovingly, *there is an old misunderstanding between you. YOU must let go of your end, in order for him to let go of his.*

I thought about this, looking at the knot of string, and within seconds the image of this man with whom I was so angry transitioned into that of a little boy. In that moment, I "saw" that his true self was innocent. He was innocent. **I was innocent.** We were hurting each other for no other reason than because we were in so many ways just human and like little children ... playing at life and making mistakes. At the soul's level, though, I knew then that this man felt true love for me. He just did not know it as he was. An immediate release happened inside me for him. **Deep and true forgiveness happened**. I forgave this man, with whom I had been so desperately angry with for so many years. It was a full, complete feeling of release, total in its sincerity, and my angel knew it. He showed me then a picture of what my life could be if I stayed. I saw myself laughing with my hair flying behind me, while I was zipping around in a speedboat. I felt a man with me, whom I could not see. But he loved me and I loved him. And I was happy, so very, very happy.

In that moment, I looked at my angel and I could see his expression softening. He said, *Trust. You must trust, Stacey. Know that you are loved and are safe. You must surrender and trust. All will be well. It is your choice …*

I made the decision in that moment to stay. The door that had been forming disappeared instantly. My angel nodded ever so slightly to me and I could see and feel that he was pleased.

You may make a wish, he said.

I replied immediately, *I want to feel JOY!*

And so shall that be, my angel said.

My angel continued to remain with me longer. *Trust,* he said over and over to me. *Surrender and Trust. Know that you are loved. Trust!* I saw then in my mind a tiny baby and my angel said, *Wrapped in swaddling … you must ride the waves of your life now without struggle.*

I could clearly see then in my mind the image of a wrapped baby floating up and down on the waves of the water.

I understood!

I deeply understood what my angel was telling me. I

felt FREE suddenly! I felt released, full of deep peace and joy, and with complete understanding of how to live my life to keep this feeling of peace. I needed to be more relaxed every day and to move with the waves of my life without struggling so.

My angel said a few more personal and private things to me, and when I felt ready, and he knew it, he ever so slowly smiled, removed his glasses, and instantly **a flash of incredible brilliant light, so immensely bright**, came shooting out of his face, eyes, and smile.

He was magnificent! The intensity and brightness of the light beaming out of him was such that I had to close my eyes.

From my angels beaming "light-force," I felt a powerful push backwards, back into my body. It was then that I realized I actually had been out of my body, floating above myself. When I opened my eyes again, I could see that the wall clock was back into its normal position. I lay on my bed, calmed and deeply settled within myself. I saw the time; it was 11:00 PM on the dot. A nurse came in just then and told me that the pulmonary doctor was traveling back to the hospital, and would see me first thing in the morning. He had recommended a sleeping pill for me. All my earlier feelings of being afraid that I would die were gone, and within a little while after receiving the sleeping pill I fell into a deep restful sleep. I was awakened early in the morning by two nurses who needed to draw my blood. While they were doing that I replayed in my mind the visit that I had with my angel. It seemed incredible to me. I believed it had happened, but still feeling weak from so much blood being lost, I was hesitant, not sure for a moment ... *Did this visit really happen?* I wondered.

The nurses that came into my room during the morning were all still wearing masks. It was not determined yet if I had some kind of foreign virus that would cause me to suffer a hemorrhage. Before long, when I was starting to think maybe the angelic visit had been really a dream, a beautiful incredible-looking black woman walked into my room. Although she wore no mask, I believed her to be a nurse. But she had no name tag on her uniform like the others. She came straight to my bed and stared down at me. I was actually so captivated by the sheer perfection of her appearance I could not speak. Her hair, eyes, and skin were of a level of beauty such as I had never before seen. She smiled at me and said, "Stacey, do you believe in God?"

I said, "YES, I do!"

"Do you believe that God can do anything, heal anything and save everything?"

"**Yes!**" I told her.

She immediately put her two hands onto my left arm and began a prayer-like statement: "Oh Jesus, beloved son of God. Thank you for sending to us your baby girl Stacey, so that we may care for her and heal her body totally. She is with us and we are with you and may no evil touch her all throughout her remaining days." She quietly said more words of prayer over me that I do not exactly remember, but her words left me feeling electrified. Any remaining doubts vanished as to whether what I had experienced the previous night was an angelic visit or a dream.

I **knew** it had been real.

This magnificent woman smiled at me, kissed me on the top of my head and left. I was so affected by her presence I was completely still. *Was that another angel?* I asked myself.

I did not know. After several minutes I realized that it did not really matter. I was fully and completely at peace.

About three hours later, my pulmonary doctor arrived. He took the seat in my room and immediately apologized that he had not been at the hospital the day before. He knew I had lost a lot of blood and said that he was scheduling, for later that morning, a bronchoscopy, a procedure to look down my throat, which hopefully would show what was causing the bleeding. I commented to him that since I had awoken, the bleeding was much reduced, but he indicated a bronchoscopy was a must.

I was moved to the ICU. Kathy had brought my suitcases over and everything of mine was in this new ICU room with me. A few hours went by before the procedure began. Immediately into it, once the doctor had the scope down my throat, he pulled the scope back up and literally ran out of the room. I was under a little anesthetic, but I could see by the looks on the technician and the nurse's faces that the abrupt end to this procedure was not normal.

Long minutes passed. The doctor never came back into my room, but the head ICU nurse did. (You know you're in serious trouble when a nurse speaks to you in the tone and manner normally reserved for three-year-olds.) *"You're going for a helicopter ride!!"* she said, as if I were heading off to an amusement park. I had no idea why this could be happening, and she did not say.

Before long, a physician's assistant came in and apologized for the doctor's departure, stating that he was on the phone at this time working to arrange my flight transport and reception at the Cleveland Clinic's Fort Lauderdale hospital. He added, "You have a huge blood clot that is covering one of your lungs and that lung has collapsed." You need to be immediately transported to our Fort Lauderdale facility and there waiting for you will be a team, headed by a cardiothoracic surgeon."

I asked, "What is a cardiothoracic surgeon?"

He replied, "Someone who specializes in both heart and lung complications."

In an hour or so a flight team from the University of Miami arrived. The pilot and the paramedic assistant came into my room and began to arrange for my immediate departure. The pilot was from France and the paramedic was from South Boston. He and I got on together right away, since I am from New Hampshire. I attended college in Boston and so we were fast friends. The pilot told me my bags could not come with me because the helicopter was a very small, jet style for fast transport and there simply was not enough room. I panicked at the idea of my bags not coming with me, as if I would never need them again. I said no loudly, insisting my bags needed to come with me. The paramedic sensed I was getting into real distress and pulled the pilot aside, saying that he would make room indeed for my bags. With that, we left to go outside.

I had no idea how bad a blood clot like mine was, but I could see clearly that the hospital staff all around me felt it was a most serious condition and they handled me with tremendous care. Eyes were wet and smiles were shaky. The jet helicopter was a dark green and to me looked like a large toy. I believe they called it "The Hornet." They loaded me up quickly and soon we took off. We flew, I noticed, low to the ground. The paramedic kept me comfortable and watched my blood pressure, signaling twice to the pilot information that seemed to bring the helicopter even lower to the ground. Not much was said to me about what might happen, but it was very clear the paramedic was watching everything. I, however, watched the Florida landscape right below pass by. Trees, traffic, homes, it all went by quickly and before I knew it, we landed on a helicopter pad near the hospital. I was transported in by ambulance. When I arrived I was greeted by a team of two doctors and three nurses. I was admitted first into a room with another young woman who immediately commented that the whole hospital floor was talking about the fact I was flown in by a medical helicopter. She was excited, and wanted to know what it was like! I honestly could not really answer as there was some more coughing up of blood and my attention was on all that this new team started to do. Shortly after I arrived another bronchoscopy was done.

The doctors that night immediately requested family come down to Florida as quickly as possible. Knowing that my entire family could not make such a long trip, not knowing what was to be or how long I would be there, I asked that my mom contact my older brother Billy, who indeed flew down immediately the next day to be with me. He stayed through the entire time, three weeks total, never leaving my side. Kathy as well came over to Fort Lauderdale and together they kept me company through long days, procedures, and surgery. While it was very stressful, not knowing what actually caused the hemorrhage, there was a strange sense of relief, to not have to work or make calls, return calls, and/or worry about the daily business. Things were taken care of for me, by my team at home, and I had an opportunity to disconnect in a way I never had before.

Over those three weeks, I read the spiritual books that I had and I felt everything would be okay. I shared with Kathy and Billy the details of my angel visit. They both totally believed me without any hesitation. Seeing that belief firsthand validated for me that I had experienced something exceptional, and in sharing it with them, they too it seemed benefited from the loving messages this visit had given me. Kathy and Billy are two people in my life that I knew beyond doubt loved and trusted me deeply. Having them accept my story unconditionally and without question led me to sense that on some level they too had been touched and maybe healed on a certain level. This belief left me with the commitment to share my story on a wider scale one day, and it gives me tremendous happiness to be able to do that here in this book. There are so many people today who need to know that they are not alone and are fully loved. It is my deepest wish that anyone reading my words here knows that my story can be their story too. Just reach UP, look within, and ask.

After about a week more in the Cleveland Clinic Fort Lauderdale, when the doctors were still unsure what had caused the hemorrhage or how best to treat it, there was a theory being floated that I might be suffering from Goodpasture's disease/syndrome. Potentially fatal, it is a rare autoimmune disease in which antibodies attack the lungs and kidneys, leading to bleeding from the lung and ultimately kidney failure. It often affects men more than women. When Dr. Stahl, my cardiothoracic surgeon, told me about this very serious possibility, I looked him in the eye and said, "I did not come here to die, doctor, I will be okay."

I did not say any more than that, but Dr. Stahl was a no-nonsense doctor. Straight to the point and very clinical, he looked at me with a directness that tried to detect any false bravado. When he did not see it, he said, "Let's hope you're right. We will, though, be taking our time on this, proceeding very slowly and carefully. We first need to remove the clot and try and get your lung to re-inflate. If it does not, we will have many issues to consider."

A team was assembled, but it was not until that next week that the procedure to remove the clot happened. It was successfully removed and my lung did re-inflate on its own. Loud cheers went up inside the surgery room, with my brother Billy actually right outside the door. When I woke up later in my room, my pulmonary doctor visited me soon after. He told me in glowing terms how beautiful my blood clot was in that it was attached so well, it would not have detached itself and traveled into my brain or anywhere, which had been their biggest fear. The consistency and make-up of the clot showed vibrant health to the body and for the most part, they were very hopeful that this whole episode was almost over.

I replied, "This clot was designed by God," adding "I think it saved my life in that it stopped the vast majority of my hemorrhage without any further loss of blood."

A little amazed at my faith in this, my doctor said, "Well, maybe you're right. For sure, it was a beauty."

The bleeding and coughing up of blood, however, started up again. Confused by this, the pulmonary team scheduled a CT scan. Now that the lung was re-inflated, the pictures clearly showed that many infiltrates were on one side of my lung, causing the hemorrhage.

The doctors did not know what to make of this. They watched me very closely, consulting everyone, everywhere, in search for answers, looking for something to help them get the bleeding to finally stop. The clinical teams assigned to me were very confused on what may have caused my condition, and after another week, when the bleeding did not stop, a biopsy surgery was scheduled. The procedure took several tiny pieces of my lung, which were sent off for pathology testing both at the University of Miami and the Cleveland Clinic in Ohio. While I was under anesthesia my cardiothoracic surgeon was deeply concerned that the bleeding needed to be stopped immediately. After several consultations with other doctors, his choice of treatment was to try 325 mg of IV steroids, or to treat me as if I did have Goodpasture's disease/syndrome. Once the IV steroids were given, Dr. Stahl stabilized me on a breathing machine and kept me unconscious for over a day and a half. They woke me when initial tests came back negative for Goodpasture's and several other possible diseases. There was no answer on why my lungs had the infiltrates, but thankfully, the steroids did their job and the bleeding stopped completely.

It took a good additional week before I was released. I could not fly home given my condition, so my brother Billy rented a car and after a few days of rest in a hotel, we slowly headed back home to New Hampshire. How wonderful my older brother Billy was through this entire episode at the Cleveland Clinic. He stayed by my side every day, helping me with small but important comforts like new tissues, clean gowns, clean towels and, whenever the craving hit me, a chocolate frappe (known as a milkshake by everyone outside of New England). I would only be able to take a couple of sips as that was all I could tolerate, but he went out whenever a craving hit me and secured one, even though we both knew I would not be able to have very much. He was a total rock for me throughout all the days of non-answers and treatment delays. With him near me I was able to remain very calm and confident in my faith that soon this whole episode would be over and we could head home.

Once home, Billy helped me with all of my unpacking, settling me in; he changed my bandages, went grocery shopping for me, and in general was very supportive. My youngest brother Michael and his wife had come during the three weeks to feed and care for my two cats. I had two beautiful animals and I had missed them terribly. They had missed me too; in fact my male cat, Bailey, had decided not to come into the house at all for over two weeks. Michael was afraid he had run off, but I lived in a renovated farmhouse, and the surrounding land, which was well over ten acres, had for all his years been his special world. I knew Bailey would come to the door as soon as I got back. And he did. Right after Billy left, I could hear Bailey at the front door meowing. He must have missed me terribly as he was an absolute mess. He smelled bad, as if he had not been cleaning himself at all, and his eyes were very sad. I remember this night so well; it was just awful to see him like this. He was always such a happy and immaculate animal. He came into the house and rushed over to me and purred so loudly. I could tell that he knew something was amiss with me. He did not immediately jump onto me, but instead he sat back and openly stared at me. My other cat, Misty, was hiding inside the house and she came out as well.

Bailey and Misty ate together and then Bailey lay next to me on the floor and proceeded to give himself a one-hour bath. When I climbed into bed, Bailey, who normally slept at the bottom of the bed near my feet, did something amazing. He gingerly tiptoed up the right side of the bed (the side my bandage and wound was on) and ever so gently positioned and laid himself down all along the right side of my body, stretching his twenty-two-pound body out completely against me, alongside my wound, placing his head directly onto my right shoulder. All I could hear was his gentle, loving purring. Bailey's head was pretty large and with his head on my shoulder like that, I could feel his soft fur on my lower chin. It felt so amazingly good. I always knew that animals are incredible loving beings, but I could not believe Bailey sensed and knew exactly where I hurt physically, and where the wound was on my body. But he did. And he stayed in this position all night. When I got up for any reason, Bailey quietly followed, giving me the most penetrating looks. It was unlike any other experience I have ever had with one of my animals and is an event I have never forgotten.

Within a few days, something even more incredible happened to welcome me back home to New Hampshire. After my third day I went outside early one beautiful morning and walked around the front side of my house. There all over the ground in front and around the backside of the house, near the tall grasses and under the trees, were **FEATHERS!!** *Dozens and dozens of feathers!* Varied colors, shapes, and sizes were spread out like a carpet all over the green grass. My first thought was that something had happened to a flock of birds, but no ... a closer look showed no evidence of injury. Gorgeous feathers, though, were all around. White feathers, gray feathers, brown, black, blue and mixed were all lying there on the grass. I was in a whirl of feelings. It took a few minutes before something inside me **"clicked"** and I started laughing and crying all at the same time.

Finally ... I connected the true meaning of all the feathers I had been seeing for so many years!

It was God, speaking to me and showing me that **HE** was near.

What JOY. Pure, unbelievable JOY I FELT!

My wish that I made with my angel had come true – I was feeling JOY – and I knew then without any doubt that God was with me, HE was inside me, HE was all around.

God is everywhere!!!

He is inside my animals, inside the trees, inside the leaves, and the grass. HE was himself the soft breeze! Everywhere, HE was everywhere and in finally knowing this, and in feeling this connection, despite how often I had believed I had known HIM before, I knew HIM now in this moment like no other. While miracles and visitations by angels are fantastic, what I felt then was a deep abiding LOVE inside my heart. I felt an enduring, everlasting love which can only come from God.

<u>I FINALLY TRULY BELIEVED!</u>

I believed then in this moment in a way that has never changed for me since.

God IS! GOD IS ALL. HE IS PURE LOVE! All I needed to do is **Trust ... *to surrender and trust ... HIM.***

Since that morning I have thought often on why "we" as humans are always separating ourselves from God. For over 2,000 years people all over the world have searched for confirmation that God is real and in our daily lives. Since the first days of creation, and throughout all generations, the truth is that God has always been with us. It is we who have separated ourselves from HIM. The mystery of where God can be found is within our own hearts. *That* is where He always has been!

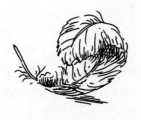

CHAPTER 5

More Miracles

I N THE DAYS AND WEEKS FOLLOWING MY RECOVERY ANOTHER small miracle occurred. My business partner, with whom I had been having such difficulty, called me to ask if we could bury the past and move on together without any further confusion or frustration. His voice, his manner was all loving, and full of heartsickness about what we had both been through. I told him I was ready to do just that and that I had already fully forgiven him and hoped he was willing to forgive me for anything I did to disappoint him. He said he could not even remember why we were so angry all the time with each other. So "the knot," the misunderstanding between us, was dissolved. And neither of us needed to do anything more than to just forgive and let it go. Which we did, and in the years following, we have kept between ourselves only good communication and cooperative spirit. While we would never be "friends," we were honorable partners. And that sometimes is all one can pray for in some of life's situations.

The balance of 2001 was a very interesting year for me. I got stronger physically, I was back to work and everything with the daily business was healthy and harmonious. We had good strong customer accounts, plenty of cash flow, and in general a feeling of tremendous ease and rhythm. I was so happy. I was fulfilling long-held desires in taking time off, spending some afternoons at the beach I love in Kennebunk, Maine, sleeping well, and enjoying every day. My life was developing deep richness.

Then on the morning of September 11, 2001, the office had a visitor walk in who started yelling about a plane having hit one of the World Trade Center towers in New York City. I felt a chill go through my body. This was only the first plane. We did not have a TV in the office, and the information startled me so much that I drove home to see what was going on. Once in the house, when I turned on the TV, the second plane had just hit Tower Two. I was stunned. I knew immediately something with this could not possibly be right. It had to be a terrorist attack of some kind. As the world watched I saw the towers come crashing down to the ground, and the beginnings of awareness happened in my mind that this could not be anything else but terrorism. The shock of these events had me on the floor praying. *Please, God, don't tell me that I agreed to stay here only for me to be witnessing now the start of World War III. It cannot be that I am here to live through that!* I was so shocked at what I was watching and all day I was numb deep inside my body. I was afraid for the country. I was afraid this was going to spiral out of control in ways no one could foresee. I was heartbroken. I prayed for answers and received no reply except a deep sense of reassurance that I would be safe and World War III would not happen.

Within the following few months, it was clear the country was going to change. Although I tried not to allow in any panic about the uncertain events and future, the daily fears caused by the constant police alerts, the news reports that big cities could be attacked at any time with dirty bombs, that bridges were vulnerable to being blown up, and in general the impression being that no one was really safe anywhere, all shook me inside. I grew more convinced, as a result, that I needed to take my life and move now into a totally new direction. I was ready for the next chapter to begin, but I did not know yet what that was.

My mom lived in Florida at this time in a wonderful small house in a retirement community. I went to visit her often. I loved the area, Vero Beach, where she lived. It was a beautiful place. Something it seemed was calling me there, some new home maybe, some new ... something, I could not yet define it, but the pull was strong.

While I was visiting with Mom one weekend, I decided with her help that I needed a long relaxing vacation, and after a lot of research made plans to travel for a ten-day trip to Anguilla. I stayed at a gorgeous resort in Anguilla with a beautiful long stretch of beach. The water was an incredible blue-green color and the resort itself was small, very well appointed, and the food fantastic. I slept, read, and swam each day and loved it. While there I was able to go deep within myself and during the long lazy afternoons, soaking up great sun, and feeling now refreshed, I realized that I was closer to knowing what it was that I wanted for myself. It was *Love*. I wanted to find love, to be loved, and to know love with a man who was perfect for me.

During one of my many strolls up and down the beach I saw one afternoon a huge heart-shaped design in the sand someone had made early that morning. On a whim, I sat in the middle of it and just lay back. I had a cozy feeling lying there and without giving in to any specific thought, after a time these words just flowed out of me: "Dear God, I know you are with me. I feel ready now after all this time to be loved and to love. I want to be with a man who loves me. Who loves me for exactly who I have been and who I am now; wanting nothing more from me than to love me, be with me and to care for me. I will accept whoever you send to me as I know he will be perfect in every way. I trust in all that you do." I said this prayer a couple of times with tears running down my face. I was ready ... truly ready to meet a man. *A husband I hoped.* And with that, I got up from the sand, went into the water, and swam for several hours. I did not think on this prayer again and I did not dwell. I just felt that as God saw fit, I would meet the right man. I was hoping deep down ... that maybe it would be soon. The month was April 2002.

During the summer of 2002, I continued to travel for the company, enjoying every day. Business trips were proving easy and customer accounts were happy. Supplies were coming in without any difficulty, and our employees were doing a fantastic job. I was visiting my mom on a regular basis and finding more and more reasons to look for a property near her home in Vero Beach. By fall, I saw down the street from where she lived a unique small house with land for horses. It was a cute and very unusual contemporary with a lot of trees around the property, and the lot itself looked snug. I loved it and decided I needed to have a realtor show it to me the next time I was down.

While visiting my esthetician for a facial during early September, I noticed a new front desk person was working there. I had an odd immediate feeling about this woman and her husband after noticing her wedding ring. It was most uncharacteristic of me to have any sense of someone else's marriage, but I had a hunch something with hers was not well, and that somehow I was going to be a part of it. I actually had a thought that I would have an affair with her husband. Such an idea was pure craziness, and it so disturbed me that I forced it out of my mind. I had never met this woman and so where these thoughts were coming from made no sense. I did not say anything on this visit, asking who she was, but a month later, in October, when I was in, I did. I asked about who this woman was and why was she not in on this day. I learned that she had decided fairly abruptly during this past June 2002 to leave her husband and family for a man she had reunited with during a high school reunion – an old boyfriend. She had, in fact, left the area and moved to Key West. My esthetician told me that when she came back to New Hampshire for a few days to see the kids, and gather more of her personal items, she would sometimes work for a day. She further told me that the woman's husband, Tom, in trying to keep the children connected and near their mother, had begun real estate classes in Florida, and with the help of a very good friend there, he was planning on working real estate for him in Vero Beach.

VERO Beach – Real Estate! I jumped out of the chair.

"I want to buy property in Vero!! I am looking right now at something near my mom's that I want to see."

She said, "You must meet Tom then; he is this woman's husband and he is simply awesome! He can help you," … then she said, "Oh, My God, I am getting goose bumps, here look!! You need to meet him, Stacey, I can just feel it, and you need to meet him soon!"

Being somewhat thrown by all this as I was not trying to make a romantic connection, I just said, "Well, uh – okay, you can just give him my name, and ask that he call me sometime. I am heading back to my mom's for Thanksgiving and want to see properties then." She agreed, but was giddy throughout the rest of our appointment.

It gets more interesting ...

My esthetician gave my telephone number to Tom. He wrote my name and number down on a piece of paper and left it on the kitchen counter, planning on calling me sometime that following week. That very weekend, his wife came home from Florida again and when she saw my name and phone number, she asked Tom how he had gotten it. When he told her she was thrilled and said, "You're going to love her, and she is great, runs her own company and is a great client of the salons. Call her, Tom ... you need to call her; she could be your first client!" Tom did not know what to make of her enthusiasm, and was not sure if the timing for a sale for him was right just then, as he had not taken his Florida exams, but he was getting ready to.

About three days later I did receive Tom's first call. He was very pleasant, spoke about Vero Beach and his plans to move there with his kids so they could be near their mom. Tom was a US Airways pilot at the time and relocating was not an issue. He could fly out to his domicile in Boston from anywhere. Lots of pilots live far away from their domicile location for work. It is very common. As he explained to me his personal situation with his wife, their soon-to-be-finalized divorce, and his plans to move to Florida, I realized he had a lot on his plate. I was actually hopeful I would find a property I did like, especially the one I had my eye on, and that maybe he could have the sale. As it turned out, his best friend from high school was the mega realtor in Vero Beach, and I had seen his signs everywhere. What a coincidence I kept thinking. *Ahem* ...

It was now around early November and my plans to head to Vero for Thanksgiving to be with my mom and my older brother Billy were fixed and I was excited. Kathy was to be there too. I love Thanksgiving; it is my favorite holiday, and being with a small crowd for a great dinner always makes me very happy. As promised in his follow-up with me, Tom always called me back exactly when he said he would, and he provided me some information on the house I had my eye on. He had also spoken to his friend Eugene, who promised him that he would show me some properties when I was in town for the holiday. Tom was due to finish his real estate classes in a few weeks and would take the Florida exam in December 2002. So the timing was actually really great. Eugene promised to show me around and hand any sale he might make with me over to Tom.

Thanksgiving arrived. The weather was wonderful and the holiday went really great. It was a perfect week and I was feeling confident that when I met Tom's friend Eugene, I would find the right house. When we first met I noticed he took a long perusal of me. He was very cordial and showed me several terrific properties, actually trying very hard to find something I really liked. As it turned out, the property I had high hopes for had some mold issues and a few other structural issues that made it unacceptable, so while disappointed, I still had a good feeling that eventually I would find something.

At the end of the first morning, after I left Eugene, he

immediately called Tom and asked him, "HAVE YOU MET STACEY YET???"

Tom said, "No, we have only spoken on the phone."

He yelled again ... "YOU HAVE GOT TO MEET HER ... SOON!"

For me, what I was focusing on regarding Tom was that he called me regularly and at the exact hour whenever he said he would. As well, it was clear we were becoming comfortable friends. He told me what Eugene said about me, but it didn't affect me at all. I mean, *what is anyone to make of that kind of a statement?* As far as I was concerned Eugene knew I was very interested in finding a home ... so maybe Tom for sure would have a first sale soon.

A FIRST SALE ... I'D SAY!

When I got back to New Hampshire, I immediately made plans to travel back to Florida for Christmas. I wanted to keep up the search for a home, and spending Christmas with Mom was something I always enjoyed. Tom was calling me by now at least two to three nights a week. He had a very soothing manner and while we spoke a bit on his divorce and the difficulties some of this created for him, overall he was a very upbeat and positive man. I like positive men; they are sometimes hard to find after a certain age. And given that he had a divorce process looming, an imminent home sale happening, as well as a new move coming up, I admired his courage and outlook on life. It was clear that his kids' welfare was most important to him, and I was thoroughly impressed by that.

Two weeks before Christmas I was scheduled to go on a business trip in the early morning out of Manchester. Rough weather and snow were expected and since I was scheduled on a US Airways flight, Tom called me the night before and indicated we might not leave in the morning. He told me about the weather pattern coming in and said he would call me in the morning to update me. As it happened, snow did arrive but it wasn't that bad just yet in Manchester. My flight was supposed to depart at 6:00 AM and we boarded. Sitting with my coffee and paper fifteen minutes before takeoff, I was pretty sure we would go. However at 6:15 AM, the pilot announced the flight was cancelled due to weather and we began to deplane. While I was still in the Jetway, my cell phone rang and it was Tom, letting me know my flight was cancelled. I laughed, saying I already knew that and was deplaning. While I was walking back to the out-side area, Tom asked since I was grounded, how about we get a coffee or something later that day? The coffee invite evolved into dinner at a local restaurant in Exeter, New Hampshire, which was about halfway between us.

I met Tom that night for the first time. My initial impressions were that he was a real nice guy. He seemed a little nervous, so we walked up and down the town's streets before heading inside the restaurant, which seemed to settle him some. During dinner I noticed that he was a good-looking man, very nice, but in no way did I feel that this was a "date," just a visit to meet someone who might help me find a home in Vero. Tom, I noticed, had a cocky side, which was tempered with a little boy spirit that made him very comfortable to be around. He was always smiling, eyes sparkling, and despite going through very difficult times he showed not one bit of fatigue. I enjoyed myself a lot, but did not consider anything more out of this night than what

I saw it as. Tom walked me out to the car and it was clear to me that he was very nervous. He leaned over to kiss me goodnight and I then left.

The next morning Tom called by 8:00 AM and asked if I had enjoyed myself. "I did," I told him. We spoke a few minutes and then we were both off to work. That night Tom called again and asked if I would meet him for dinner later in the week. I actually had a meeting in Massachusetts that Thursday and so we made plans to meet in Woburn, Massachusetts, at 6:00 PM. When I arrived in the parking lot, Tom was waiting in his car. When he came over to my car, I could see he was holding something behind his back. When he pulled it out, there was a long-stemmed single red rose and a Tupperware bowl full of homemade chicken soup. On the soup cover it said "Merry Christmas." I was a little shocked by this as I had not expected it, nor did I expect anything like a long-stemmed rose, but I accepted both with a smile, as suddenly I had a good feeling inside me standing there next to this tall, very nice man.

We went inside the Mexican restaurant, sat back, relaxed, and took our time ordering. The first hour went by easily, then the next. Our conversation was very comfortable, with a lot of smiles and light laughter. By the time we were nearly finished with dinner and coffee, I turned from having been looking down at something, and as I looked up again at Tom, it was as if I had been hit by a truck. **BOOM!** Right between the eyes, this intense feeling just came over me. Writing about it at this moment still brings tears to my eyes. **I KNEW.** I just knew in that moment, *here is my husband*. Those thoughts were exactly what I heard inside my head. Here is the man God has found for me ... my future husband. Knowing this ... Tom was all beauty, light, and love. All these things I could have hoped, but did not ask for. All I prayed for was a man who would love me for who I was, and I knew in that moment, deep down into my very soul, Tom was that man. I was actually a little staggered and Tom looked at me a little funny, but said nothing. But in looking at me then, Tom just slowly smiled and together we just sat there silent, smiling at each other. *He was here ...* he was sitting right next to me and he was mine. Over and over, I thought these thoughts, and over and over, I felt waves of joy going through my body, like nothing I had ever felt before in my life with any man. *I was home finally ...* and no words needed to be spoken about this knowing, we just both "knew." It was about 11:15 PM when the wait staff came quietly over to our table and told us we had to leave as they were closing up the restaurant. Tom and I had no idea what time it was just then, and we burst out laughing. We had closed the restaurant! When Tom walked me to the car I felt like I was walking on air, and I thought Tom looked like he was too. My life from that moment on has never been the same, and before Tom closed my car door, I made sure he knew that was exactly how I felt ...

Every night following this night, Tom called me. While I was in Florida for Christmas, Tom phoned each day, two to three times, and then one morning as my Mom was handing the wireless phone over to me, she said, "This man is not going to make it to New Year's without needing to see you – mark my words."

I was smiling when she said that because I could feel that Tom would in fact come down very soon. He still had work travel to finish, and Christmas to complete with his kids, but I just knew he would come down to Vero Beach, and in fact he did just that. He hopped on a jump seat down to Florida on New Year's Day to see me. And we have been together almost every day, of every week, except for Tom's deployments, and business travel, ever since.

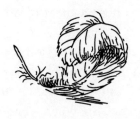

CHAPTER 6

Tom at My Side – My Stem Cell Transplantation

AND SO, ON MANY LEVELS, MY JOURNEY BEFORE MY MAR-riage and life with Tom, even my experience with cancer, is in a way Tom's journey too. Never after marriage are two souls who love each other truly separate again. And I think on some mystical level this truth, that we were "meant" to find each other and be together in this life as man and wife, Tom and I knew was true for us even in the early months after we first met. While I had had very startling spiritual experiences during my life before and after meeting Tom, he too had a few premonitions about me, before we met. Subtle signs … things Tom never really knew what to make of. One of them being that Tom would hear (out of the blue) the name "Stacey," spoken out loud in the air around him. Tom said that he did not ever have experiences like this, except in the outright hearing of my name, and he would hear it most often in the quiet of the cockpit, often before a flight take-off. Tom said he would turn and look around, thinking someone behind him had said this name out loud. But no one was ever there. He knew the other pilot had not spoken it, but yet he heard the name clearly – "Stacey." So, when we met, a tiny ping went off inside him. He was not actually consciously aware of it at first, but in a short while, he connected the dots. And of course, Tom is the man my angel showed beside me in the speedboat, with my hair whipping behind. We have had many wonderful boat rides like this together, Tom and I.

This heavenly coordination of meeting Tom, him for me, and me for him, is one of the most beautiful gifts my illness has taught me to trust in. God has the final say in how everything in one's life turns out, even if along the way beforehand, unwise choices are made and sometimes a soul may feel he or she is traveling down the wrong side of the street. Listening for guidance, trusting when forks arrive or new paths are presented in front of us, no matter how scary at first they seem, we are always carefully being led to our highest good. Reaching this type of spiritual vision or insight does not happen overnight, but trusting in the goodness of God everyday means that you can relax and know that in time all things will work out. Today, in our life and marriage there is a calmness and a serenity for Tom and me, as well as a deep knowing that together we are two halves of one whole, stronger together than apart – no matter what. But, in the weeks leading up to my transplant, Tom and I were still struggling with the unknowns, and Tom's arrival at a place of assurance that all would be well did not happen easily.

As I prepared for the upcoming transplantation, I had

four amazing brothers who all were hoping that they would be my stem cell donor. As the time drew near for the blood test results to come in, each of them called me beforehand and told me how much they wanted to be "the one." I cannot express the gratitude and unconditional love that I felt for them, because while I always knew my brothers loved me, I had no idea until then just how deeply they did. But even with that incredible security that their love gave me, there was the knowledge for Tom and me that if none of my brothers were a match, my chances of survival were not good. There is a time period during a "blast" phase for some patients, myself being one, when the cancer must be stopped. It has to be stopped and killed quickly through very aggressive total body irradiation and very strong chemotherapy, *or else.* Unlike specific and targeted radiation for some tumor-based cancers, leukemia is a blood cancer that is throughout the body. And when it becomes aggressive, it kills. Some types of leukemia if caught early can be managed and controlled very well with medications like Gleevec. Mine was developed well beyond this point. The only chance for me to live was a bone marrow stem cell transplant.

A stem cell transplant is a fascinating procedure. It had been explained to me in simple but beautiful terms. The bone marrow is made up of stem cells. Leukemia is cancer of the blood, and when in a blasting stage, the stem cells of the patient must be completely eradicated in order that new healthy stem cells, from a donor, can be implanted, allowing the patient to have a strong chance of survival. But the procedure for a transplant is still a dangerous procedure today. It takes the patient to within an inch of their life because all of their bone marrow/stem cells must be dead before the transplant of healthy donor stem cells can be provided and accepted by the body. The transplant procedure itself happens immediately once the patient's radiation and chemotherapy have done their job, but there is still great danger should any type of delay happen with the donor or the donor's stem cell collection. The window for transplant is very, very brief. A patient has no immune system following total body radiation and chemotherapy. The body is like an empty shell, just waiting for the new cells. And the waiting period is less than twenty-four hours, or the patient will die without any possible medical way for them to be saved.

The body though is miraculous, and once the donor stem cells are received through the procedure, which is actually done intravenously, the new stem cells march off instantly inside the body knowing exactly where to go, which is inside the bone marrow itself. While this sounds simplistic and beautiful, which it definitely is, the patient is physically devastated. It takes weeks and weeks to slowly recover. Transplant patients are in a hospital room and on a floor that is separated within the hospital, curtained off with plastic; all equipment inside the room is covered with plastic. The nurses, doctors, and family all must be masked and gloved while visiting. I can recall when I first was in my room feeling like I was in a capsule in some deep cavern at NASA, waiting to be shot into space. It was very surreal, this environment: foreign, totally clinical, but **safe**. The room was safe! And when you go through a transplant, understanding just how important these precautions are means everything. It is like living in a cocoon. It takes a very long time for the immune system to recover, and to this day, three years into it, my immune system still struggles. It remains a little above the 50% levels the doctors would like it to be at. But, I am alive!

I am so fortunate that my younger brother Tim was a match for me, almost a perfect, identical DNA match actually. He had himself in the years prior to my operation been improving his body through exercise and a diet of reduced fats and carbohydrates. While this is not always needed, it certainly does not hurt. The doctors and nurses told Tom that his stem cells were just about perfect. He and I believe that in some miraculous way, he was preparing, without any conscious knowledge, so that I could be saved through his stem cell donation. It is a beautiful experience to have a brother do this for you – to donate his cells, for a part of his inner cell DNA body to become you. Tim literally saved my life.

When the testing of my brothers was going on and we did not know who would be the one, or even if one of them would match, Tim was actually the last brother I imagined I would match. But, as we went through this experience together, I got to know him in a much deeper way than I had before and while we may not look a whole lot alike, we actually on the inside, our personality and temperaments, are very similar. During my transplant procedure, Tom sat in the background of my hospital room allowing Tim to be right next to me on my left side. My right arm was used for the IV that would deliver the stem cells. Days prior, Tim had stayed in a hotel next door, with his wife, Deb, to ensure that he was safe, sound, and near me for when the doctors wanted to collect his stem cells, which was the morning of my afternoon transplant.

As Tim's stem cells were delivered into the room I was surprised to see that the stem cells inside the glass container looked just like a strawberry daiquiri. The color was exactly the same. Tim smiled with pride when they arrived and told me that his clinical team indicated to him that during his stem cell collection, there were no imperfections in his stem cells, and he was thrilled by that. The procedure began easily. With his soft warm golden brown eyes shining confidence and hope for me, Tim held my left hand throughout the entire procedure. While there was no pain whatsoever, I was, however, very tired from the four days of total body radiation and the very strong chemo. Tim could feel that tiredness from holding my hand, so he smiled at me, leaning in to speak quietly to me during the entire procedure. What a feeling it was. I knew beforehand that this experience for Tim and me would connect us in a way that was new to our relationship. But this feeling, the bond that began to be formed between us, was much more palatable to me than I had thought it would be. It was amplified because Tim, himself, was so intensely proud of what he was doing for me, and his love for me was such, and his intellectual respect for the medical transplant science so profound, that it evoked from him, into me, immense strength. His force of will was tremendous and it helped me in so many ways. During the transplant Tim's focus was uninterrupted; he beamed hope and wellness through his face and eyes into mine. It was as though Tim was transmuting new life into me alongside his body's own stem cells. I could feel his sincere intention while he was holding onto my hand. He squeezed it several times, infusing me with courage. Suddenly, about three-fourths of the way into the procedure, I felt an indescribable thrill run up and through my entire body. I closed my eyes and focused on this feeling, smiling the whole time.

Tim asked, "What is it?"

I said, "I can't say exactly, but what a feeling!"

After a few more seconds, I could almost hear an inner singing ... and realized that what I was sensing was *new life!* I said to Tim, "Now I know how women who have birthed babies feel." He smiled and nodded almost like he knew too ... that this was the feeling I was having. He on some inner dimension was sharing that feeling with me. It continued ... there was such a rush, of sensation, of new life being born inside me. "This is a miracle, Tim. I had no idea ... but it is a true miracle." Tim just smiled his special sweet smile and said, "It is, and you're going to do great."

In those moments, Tim's cells were in fact saving my life, and on some level, I could feel my body's thanks and pure happiness for that. **How incredible ...**

This beautiful feeling that I was experiencing was a crescendo of sorts as to the difficult and restless days leading up to my admission into the hospital. While I was confident that the outcome would be positive, there was a moment when I could have made the wrong decision to not move forward with the transplant. So much of one's life is forever changed as a result of a transplant. It is daunting really to even think about. In the weeks leading up to the transplant I had to meet with my oncology doctor several times. During one of the last visits, I needed to sign a pile of standard "consents" allowing the stem cell procedure to occur. I noticed on one of the last pages a "consent of understanding" regarding what my life, during the first year of recovery, would entail. Reading, I was stunned to see words like "find a new home or shelter for twelve months for all pets, no plants in the home, no visitors except family, no going outside unless masked and heading to the hospital. Total and complete in home care for one year, no going outside to work in the garden or walking barefoot, no live flowers, dirt or anything from the outside; for one full year. The home needed to be thoroughly professionally cleaned. All family members must use hand sanitizers continually. No receipt of food not prepared in the home, no drinking of non-purified water," on and on. What stood out for me was the inability to leave the house for **ONE YEAR**! Give up my beloved **PETS**!

After reading all of this, I put the pen down, crossed my arms, and glared at Dr. Antin. I said to him, "This is totally unacceptable. I have a company to run. There is no chance I will agree to this and forget about me giving up my cats. **NO WAY!**" I can recall that a few seconds passed and without flinching, like a laser beam with eyes dead-locked on mine, Dr. Antin said calmly, "that's fine, but in six months you will be dead. You will go home and within three months you will take to your bed, and you will never get up again. You will suffer badly and you will be gone *if you're lucky* in six months."

The seconds passed while we stared at each other. I thought to myself then, *I have angered him.* I know now, today, that I had **scared** him. Patients do refuse to be transplanted for various reasons. I think in that moment Dr. Antin believed I was potentially one of them. By this visit, he knew I was completely devoted to my company and that I was capable of being headstrong. But while I may be headstrong, I am not reckless. After a few minutes, I slowly picked up the pen, pulled the paper back in front of me, and signed. Dr. Antin did not move a muscle until I completed the final few pages of consent. When I did he smiled a beatific smile and said, "Thank you."

I asked, "Will you be able to save my life, doctor?"

Without a second's hesitation he said to me, "Yes, but you're going to do everything, and I mean *everything* that I tell you to do, especially during the first year of recovery."

I said then, very quietly, "I cannot give up my cats. I just cannot."

Dr. Antin paused before answering and said, "You will not be able to pick them up and hold them for a long time and you will never again, in your life, be able to clean their cat boxes. And the cat boxes must not be anywhere near you."

I said with total relief that this would not be a problem. The house is large and their boxes are way down in the basement.

He replied, "That's fine; you wouldn't be going down into the basement for the next year either."

I remember that I smiled at Dr. Antin then as the worst part of the tension had passed. I said quietly, "I promise to be a good patient." Dr. Antin ended this visit with me by telling a story I never forgot, emphasizing the fact that being a "good patient" was imperative. He said that both young and old can get leukemia and while young people tend to recover from the transplant very well, it is in the year-long recovery that patients can get into serious trouble. He told the story of a twenty-five-year-old young man who did great throughout the transplant, but after a few months at home grew irritated by the confinement. He loved to go out and get donuts, and so he did. He went into his car unchaperoned and drove himself a few times off to get donuts and coffee. After the third time in one week, he drove his car straight into a tree and died before the paramedics arrived. His immune system had crashed as his exposure outside, even for a brief time, drinking and eating foods not prepared at home, caused a serious bacterial infection, which killed him swiftly. Dr. Antin's message was clear to me. "We can do miraculous things with leukemia today, be we cannot prevent a patient's own stupidity from doing them in." I vowed then I would not be one of them.

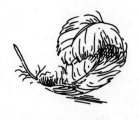

CHAPTER 7

Faith Everlasting

VERY PATIENT WHO HAS EVER BEEN IN THE HOSPITAL FOR ANY length of time knows the sounds a hospital room and hallway make. Beeping noises, hissing sounds the distant ringing of phones, machines being dragged from one room to another; it just goes on and on sometimes. These noises were soothing at times because they became so familiar, and at other times they were intensely annoying. Always though for me they triggered memories. Memories of the lovely life that I had lived with Tom, and memories of other dreams that just would never be. As I sat back in my bed one Saturday morning, into my third week of transplant recovery in December 2009, I knew that I was still mentally foggy from all that I had been through. Tom was with me as he always was, leaning back on the long bench cushion in my hospital room. His eyes were tired and he had dark circles underneath. He had driven down from New Hampshire to be with me again that entire day, a good two-hour drive each way, when there was traffic, which often there was. There are many ways in life that a man can show you how much he loves you. For Tom and me we had met each other at a point in our lives where we just were both past the need for constant, small romantic gestures to keep ourselves connected. Years earlier, we had decided as a couple to keep Christmas gifts to each other simple or none at all. A beautiful dinner, maybe a trip somewhere, but presents were just not necessary. Tom would spontaneously bring home roses for me and always for our anniversary and my birthday. Together we had pretty much all that any two people could want. We had a beautiful home, nice furnishings, and appliances in the kitchen, and sufficient toys in the yard like a boat and snowmobile, the kids were grown with Jeff almost out of college; in general, our personal needs and wants were very few.

As Tom, sleepy eyed and a little slumped, gazed at me, all I could see within him was the pain experienced by a man who could not make this awful experience for his wife, his love, go away. It was not within his power to make it disappear, from what had been such an amazing day-to-day life together. I could see that this man, my husband, who was so used to being in full control of everything in his life, from flying multimillion-dollar aircraft, to organizing flights for formation, to being in full control of his own plane, his crew, and his destiny, up until this point, was feeling totally out of control for the first time in his life. And I wanted so much for this pain within Tom to resolve.

Sometimes though, there is nothing that can be said to make any unpleasant situation better. Tom would sit and witness me go through the pain of procedures, bad IVs not taking easily, vomiting, not being able to get up to go to the bathroom, the constant monitoring of vital signs by technicians, the constant inflow of nurses, doctors, OR staffers, wheelchairs, and on and on. Drugged, I was having an easier time of it most days than he was. I could barely feel anything, but always like a whisper, I knew what Tom was feeling.

There was not a day that went by while I was sick that Tom did not greet me or say goodbye to me without calling me "beautiful." "Good morning, Beautiful," he would say with a smile. And he made me feel beautiful not because he would say the word, but because he said it ... *with such feeling.* Tom and I did not depend on each other to make us feel confident in ourselves. We were and are two confident people. Calling me "Beautiful" was his special term of endearment and I knew he meant it in every way.

Before being admitted into the hospital I had decided I did not want to watch my wonderful thick hair fall out in chunks. I discussed with Tom how I would feel most comfortable handling this part of the preparation process for the surgery. So we decided to have a head shaving party at home. During it, Tom, along with Jo my hairdresser, helped me shave off my hair. Joining us were the members of my family, and a few friends with whom I was most comfortable, who would celebrate this moment of full acceptance for me of what was to come in the saving of my life. Throughout my many years, my hair had been a crowning glory for me. It was always shiny, thick, and very beautiful. Tom loved my hair as well. So, in preparing myself as a woman to be rid of it completely ... this was in truth the first authentic step in exercising my faith, regarding my cancer and that I could be "more," even without this asset I had relied on all through my years. *I needed and wanted to be courageous.* And I thought to myself before the party that there is no greater test for a woman to express her true courage than to accept herself totally and utterly bald.

It was a night I promised myself that I would approach with bravery, no matter what. I would not allow myself to cry or be embarrassed by my family and friends seeing me bald. *No, that would not happen.* I had a reservoir of strength and faith built over years of prayer to sustain me and *I would not fall down.* I had never been a vain woman and I did not have energy now to waste on foolish emotions. I prayed for the inner strength I knew was there. I would not look back ... I would not.

As Jo began to shave my head, I could see in the eyes of my family the early twinge of surprise, as my hair began to fall. Tom was standing beside me and I think he may have noticed some of that too. So he asked Jo if he could help, and she immediately handed the shaver over to him. Tom began gently to shave the remaining parts of my hair off. Although he was smiling at everyone while doing it, I later learned from Jo (a full two years later) that Tom's hand shook quite a bit while he was shaving my head. After all my hair was gone, I smiled at everyone and while I could see everyone was okay ... there was a feeling of mild shock circulating in the room. I knew it was not because they did not like the way I looked ... it was because I looked so different.

After a few words of support from everyone I took a moment to be alone in my master bedroom bath. I looked at myself in the mirror. I felt while standing there, looking at myself, that another door to my past was forever closed. It was like hearing a door slamming shut. I never expected that. Within a few minutes Tom came quietly in to stand beside me. He looked at me in the mirror and smiled. "You look beautiful," he said, and in his eyes I could see he truly meant it. He enjoyed the way I looked, he loved my face, and my not having my lovely hair did not affect his feelings for me as a woman at all. I could see that clearly. I was so … *relieved!* I did not really think I had given this insecurity much consideration beforehand … about how Tom would feel about me. My thoughts had been about how I would see myself. But here in my bathroom, minutes after my hair was completely shaved off, I was in the arms of the most important person in my life, and he simply did not care about my hair being completely gone. **Wow!** Together, Tom helped me to tie on my first headscarf, and looking back into the mirror, *I knew I would kick this cancer's butt.* Tom hugged me tight, and together we walked back out to our guests and towards what was next to come in our lives.

I had with me in the hospital next to my bed at all times one of my favorite spiritual books, White Eagle's *Heal Thyself.* I would pick this book up and select any page, and the words there would comfort me immediately. Sometimes I would read or share a paragraph with Tom. Always, it would bring me to that sound place where I felt once again very secure in the knowledge that all would be right with my life, and with Tom's, and together we would pull through without fail.

Much of my memory today of that month's recovery, immediately following transplant, while still in the hospital has a dreamlike quality to it. Some parts are vivid to me, and other parts are indistinct. During most days, while I was aware of the happenings going on all around me, I was on other levels not fully aware. I would wake up and see my brothers sitting next to me, smiling. Often, I would be too tired for any long visits. Days flowed one into the other and my sense of time was completely distorted. I would try to work a little bit and stay in touch with the office, but for the most part, they were running things without me. This was a time when everything in my life, around me and beside me, was only about me and me getting better.

Towards that, I would dream. To blunt pain, to cut off feelings of being out of control in my life, I would often just look at Tom while he was snoozing in the hospital chair beside me, and travel back in my mind to the incredible vacations and trips we had taken together. An image of Tom sliding into our hot tub in our large gorgeous guest room at the Ventana Hotel in California would appear. I could hear his laughter and the splashing noises he would make. In my mind I could smell the trees and flowers that were on the walkway all around the property and the immense beauty of the Pacific Ocean when we ate at the restaurant across the street, which had a part of their dining room over-hanging by a wide bit the wild ocean below, offering a full view of the water crashing on the rocks below. I could recall completely the smell of the horses that we rode together through Big Sur and the warmth of the sun on my face. Tom does not really like horses but he will ride them with me, because while I am not a good rider, I love horses and any chance I can get to be on one, he will do it with me. We rode horses on our honeymoon in Puerto Rico too.

I would recall often our wedding day and how beautiful it all was. Tom and I had wanted to elope, but after giving it a lot of thought we decided to have a very small gathering of twelve with us at the hotel were we stayed in Fajardo, Puerto Rico. It was one of the most beautiful days of my life. Everything, from the roses, to the gardens, to the food, to our hotel room, everything was spectacular. I wanted to remember every single minute of my wedding and to do that I had decided I needed to release all the details to my wedding planner, who did an unbelievable job. It was Perfection. Everything was total perfection. While lying back in my hospital bed I was able to recall every footstep down the aisle, the look in both Christina and Jeff's eyes, and Tom's loving regard as he took my hand. Crystal clear were these memories and they held me together through every single second of those long hours in the hospital when I would sit and not be able to carry on a conversation, while watching Tom ... watch me.

When we finally got back home to New Hampshire, in late December 2009, we had a long list of medical dos and don'ts and it was absolutely necessary to have caregiver help for me. My loving stepdaughter Christina carried most of the burden of daily care for me, on those days when Tom needed a break, or when he started to go back to work. She separated out the multitude of drugs I needed to take, morning, afternoon, and night. She helped Tom do the grocery shopping, she took care of the cats, she did everything that I needed but most of all, Christina was "with" me in spirit every moment. My fondest memory of both Christina and Jeffrey were the deep loving looks that they would give me. It is just difficult being sick. No matter how spiritual and confident one is in one's place in God's hands, being sick totally sucks: the nausea, the vomiting, and the needing help in and out of the bath, sometimes on and off the throne, eating, walking, and climbing stairs. It was a 24/7 care situation and it went on for a full year. It abated near the end of the first year for sure, but it was constant. The other constant was setbacks and revisits for long weeks back into the hospital, all throughout 2010.

However, blessings never ceased. In the years prior

to my illness, Tom and I used to be drawn to the idea of and search for a lakefront property. When I was a child, my family had a camp on Lake Winnipesaukee and every summer we spent weekends and long weeks up there on that huge beautiful lake. Tom loves to boat and fish and together we would just head out in search of that special place we could have as a weekend home for summers. We did not need anything too big; we just wanted to find a cozy place on one of the lakes. We could find nothing. We searched, we drove, we looked online, but year after year, we could not see anything we thought we could afford or that fit the combination of "must haves." We wanted neighbors, but not on top of us. We wanted lakefront, but not at the expense of being squeezed on top of our neighbors like sardines; we wanted to be within an hour from home so Tom could head back to work without too much driving; and most important, we wanted something the kids would love. Nothing ever appealed until one day in October 2009, just before learning I would need a transplant, I was surfing online, searching once again for lakefront, when I noticed a new set of listings, on a lake I had never heard of before. It was close enough to our home and yet also to Lake Winnipesaukee, so knowing the area, I was excited. I called the realtor and told her of our long years of looking for property, and incredibly, we had never heard of this lake I was seeing now. We agreed to meet, with her telling me that all around this lake area there were other smaller, lesser known lakes too, that also had homes for sale. I was intrigued. We met a few days later and together in her slightly beat-up car, we drove around and visited several properties in the order she chose. Some had potential I thought. The prices were not too high, a few were of course, and several had nice waterfront, with very motivated sellers. I was hopeful, but did not yet see anything that I thought both Tom and I would love.

I was getting a little tired after several hours of driving around and asked if we could call it a day. Zana, my realtor, asked if we could pop into one more listing she had on her plan, and since it was close enough to where we were, I said yes. When we arrived at the home, it had a lot of the "must haves"; it had a long dirt road leading up to it, with few homes around. Nice privacy I could see. It also sat on a point, and had a lot of waterfront, but not a clear view as Tom would have hoped for. The property was surrounded by pine trees and birches. While you could certainly see water, it was peek-a-boo. Here, there, and a little over everywhere, but no big wide open view as I knew Tom would have wanted. As we walked up to the house, I could hear the birds chirping, which I love. It was a fairly simple house, brand new, and had been on the market for quite a long time, without much of a history of showings.

I nodded and looked and listened to Zana as she recited the house's good points when as we approached the front door and as she was reaching for her keys, there on the doormat I saw a long Black Feather! I gasped and swooped down to pick it up. **A FEATHER!** There, right there, was this beautiful shiny perfect black feather, with no other feathers around anywhere that I could see. There it was waiting for me, right there on the doormat. Zana looked at me a little strangely, but of course, if I was happy – well, that could mean only good things for her! We walked into the house and it was a well-done lake home with nice high vaulted ceilings made of knotty pine, the wood was all good, not overdone, not underdone, a good solid second home. I felt Tom would really like it. The price was high, maybe a little too high given the market and our budget, but we could deal with that later. I held onto the feather and thanked Zana, ready now to head home. I told Tom about the home that weekend and together we drove up to see it. As we drove up to it, Tom went very silent. He did not move a muscle for long minutes as we sat in the car, staring all around. He turned and looked at me with total wonderment in his eyes, loving everything he was seeing, and we had not yet even gotten out of the car. It was then that I showed Tom the feather. He smiled at me thinking I was a little bit funny. He was looking at the amount of lakefront there was and here I was showing him *the feather*. We got out of the car and began to walk around. Misty tears were coming to Tom's eyes. It was love at first sight for him. He was enthralled. We stayed on the property for about an hour, went down to the dock, walked on the deck, and realized with deep certainty that this was the home we had been searching for.

The next day we spent a good deal of the morning talking about the house. We nicknamed it "Blue Wave." Tom wanted to go back and look at it again, so we did. We stopped along the way at the local diner and picked up a couple of sandwiches. We had two cloth deck chairs in the trunk and when we arrived back at the house, we took the sandwiches and the chairs and sat out on the deck of the home, and just tuned into everything all around. "Could we do it?" we asked each other. "Can we afford it?" Well, at the current price not that easily, but it was not totally out of the question. We knew we did not want to be strapped on payments. Tom hates bills, hates having anything not paid exactly on time as he does not like financial stress at all. I don't either, but in building a company from scratch, I was used to dealing with cash flow issues so for me, if there is a will, there is always a way. It just sometimes takes a lot of time and careful thought. So, we talked, we ate, we walked around again and then we left – committed to figuring it out.

Once back home, I called Zana and we made an offer substantially below the asking price. It was a base point that we felt comfortable with, and so we made the offer. A prompt "no thank you" came back immediately. *Hmmm.* "Okay," I said to Tom, "we have to wait. I have the feather, which tells me that this is the right home, maybe just not yet the right time."

Tom was a little frustrated, but he accepted it because going any higher in price at this point was beyond his comfort zone, and so we just agreed for now to let it go. The market then was unfavorable to sellers and knowing it was on a quiet, little-known lake, we held out the hope that maybe it would work out somehow at a later point. It was about ten days later that Tom and I would learn from Dr. Steinberg I would need a donor transplant. So feather or not, the lake house was wiped completely out of our minds.

Following my stem cell transplant and after having been home for a couple months, on a sunny but cold Sunday morning in late February, Tom looked up at me, smiled, and said the words, "Blue Wave."

I slowly smiled back and said, "Oh, yeah."

Tom continued to smile at me and asked how I was feeling. It was for me a "good day." I was not having too much of a bad time with nausea and my spirits were good. Tom said, "Can I bundle you up and take you for a drive?"

For the most part, my only outings were confined to our weekly trips back to Dana Farber for follow-ups, so the idea of getting masked and gloved and going for a drive in a heavy winter coat, while a bit of work, held appeal if what Tom wanted to do was visit the lake house. We had not spoken of it at all in the long months that had just passed. I was not certain if I was strong enough, but Tom felt I could do it. I would not get out of the car, but maybe we could both sit and look around ... he was asking. I said "yes," and like the little boy that he truly is inside, Tom jumped up to get everything ready. Once in the car, we noticed that trees along the highway held tons of snow and it was visually beautiful. Most of the people who have homes on the lake were gone for the winter so when we arrived, it was intensely quiet and as a result, the beauty of the surroundings for me was amplified. I thought it was stunning. As beautiful as it was with the water and sunlight through the trees when we last saw it, this too was magnificent. Tom loved it as well and while I stayed inside the car, he got out and walked around. When he came back he looked me in the eyes and said, "Let's make this work. We deserve it and I want for you to have it. I want us to have it," ... and he closed with his trademark, "Are you with me, girl??" When I said "YES, I am with you," he closed with **"Roger that ... let's get on it!"**

We headed back and when we arrived home, I went to take a nap, allowing Tom to spend some time alone in his thoughts. I had learned by this point in our marriage that Tom does best when he has time to consider things alone within himself. Later that afternoon we took out paper and pen and began to crunch the numbers. Months had passed, and the house had not sold. We loved it, and we wanted it, and so a compromise needed to be reached on the price. We agreed we were willing to pay more than our previous offer. We decided how to do it and settled together on a max price beyond which we would walk away. This was the hardest part because we loved the house so much, and by now we really felt like it was meant to be ours, that walking away due to several thousands of dollars just felt wrong. But math is math and our financial goals and the stresses about money, which had so victimized much of my life in business, would not intrude or become a part of our personal life, so a line had to be drawn. And together we drew it, and agreed if we could not get the house at our max, we would accept and walk away.

As it happened, when we made our new offer, there was one small counter and we were able to accept. Thrilled, we began the mortgage closing process. About midway through the process, I had a setback whereby I needed to be readmitted into the hospital for two and a half weeks, in May 2010, for draining of both of my lungs and my heart, due to excess fluid. While the drains were not an overly painful process, I had during this hospital stay a terrible incident occur with my heart the night following my heart drain, which had me in racking, screaming pain. It was around midnight when the cramping and spasms in and around my heart started with such an incredible intensity that in short minutes I was withering on the bed, with sweat pouring down my body. The floor nurses all started to come into my room frantic to stop my pain. The doctor on the floor began to administer IV morphine, but after the first rush of warmth from the drug, the pain started up again almost immediately. Over and over the nurses and the doctor gave me shots of morphine, but it did not work. Within an hour a cardiac doctor from the ER came up to see me. I was lying on the bed, my body drenched in sweat, the bed sheets twisted in my hands from the incredible pain the spasms were causing me. I looked at this doctor and saw his mouth drop open as he reviewed the condition I was in, as well at the monitor next to the bed. He asked with a loud shout, **"How long has she been like this?!"** I don't remember any of the nurses' answers – I just looked at the doctor and pleaded, **"Please, please 'knock me out'!!"** Thankfully, he must have because it was early morning when I woke up next, without any more pain at all. What a horrible night that was and one I hope to never relive.

The lake house closing happened at our home about a week after I was discharged. With everyone masked and gloved it was a quick thirty-minute closing and then Tom and I had our keys to Blue Wave. We were ecstatic, and we still feel this way, even more today, about this house that is now our permanent home.

In the first few months we went up to the lake every weekend, getting the new furniture settled in and the boat launched, etc. I had to rely mostly on Tom, as I did not have any energy to move things, but he took care of it all and in about four weeks, I could sit out on the deck, while masked, and enjoy the outdoors. The sounds of the lake were thrilling for me and I was so happy each time we were there.

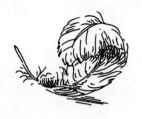

CHAPTER 8

A Medical Setback

U NBEKNOWNST TO ME, TROUBLE WAS AGAIN BREWING INSIDE
my body. I had been trying very hard to do three to
four hours a few days a week of work for the company. Emails mostly but calls too. While many daily admin-
istrative aspects were being handled by others, I was still
the CEO/President and certain business issues required
my direct attention and decisions. I was continuing
weekly visits to Dana Farber, but I also had a home care
nurse who would come by frequently and take my vitals,
clean and inspect my port, and in general keep tabs on
my overall health. Somehow though, my homecare nurse
and the nurses at Dana missed signals that I was getting
ill. Post-surgery recovery for transplant patients is fraught
with ups and downs, sometimes no more meaningful than
the patient just needing more rest, but at other times much
more serious. This was the case with me. On the weekend
of July Fourth that first summer up at the lake house, and
during dinner, I began to feel quite funny. My lips were

turning an odd color and I was very faint. Even though it was very warm that I night, I caught a chill. I ended up heading into bed by 7:00 PM, missing the fireworks and sleeping most of the next day. When back home at our primary house, that first night, I was chilled a bit again and so I took a bath. I awoke later in the night at 3:00 AM with a 103.5° fever. Tom had an early call into work and I did not want to wake him, so I crept downstairs and went back to sleep on the couch. I knew the fever was not a good sign, but I was *tired of always being so tired*, and so I did not wake Tom as I should have. A 103.5° fever for a transplant patient is very serious indeed, needing immediate medical attention without fail. When Tom woke at 4:30 AM and saw me on the couch, he asked why I was downstairs. When I told him of my fever the night before, he immediately went down into the lower level of the house and called Christina to come up that instant from her apartment near Boston, Massachusetts. I had fallen back to sleep when he came back into the living room and he did not wake me to tell me she was coming. My fever had come down by that time, so for myself, I thought there was no real concern. I woke up again about 7:30 AM, to the sounds of keyboard typing. When I turned, sitting there at the kitchen table smiling at me was my beautiful girl.

"How are you feeling?" she asked.

"I don't know," I replied.

Christina told me with a firm look that her dad had instructed her to have me immediately contact Dr. Antin about the fever. I was hesitant to do this as I knew how busy Dr. Antin was, but Christina was very direct about what Tom had said, so I did contact Dr. Antin by email. I described my symptoms over the past few days of fatigue, my lips changing color, etc., and on the fever of 103.5° just that night, and his reply came quickly back, **"Get down here immediately!!"**

With that unequivocal answer Christina helped me to gather my things and we left the house in short order. On the drive down, I was feeling pretty good and kept saying how all this concern seemed like it might be a bit of an over-reaction.

When we arrived at Dana Farber's waiting room, as usual it was packed with patients. Christina checked me in and I sat down to wait. Within five minutes, however, I started to shiver. At first it was a chill, but quickly it turned into much, much more, with uncontrollable shivering, my teeth actually chattering louder and louder. Christina jumped up and ran over to the nurses' station informing them of what was happening. Two nurses who knew me well came over to see me and in seconds, one went off to secure a wheelchair and the other headed off to secure warm blankets. Christina held onto me tightly and tried to steady me until they got back. In less than three minutes both were back and I was bundled up in the warm blankets and immediately wheeled into the private clinical area for infusions and exams.

While in this room my body began to decline very quickly and it was decided to transport me immediately into the emergency ICU area. Christina called Tom and he headed straight down, joining me in less than two hours. During that time, the doctors had me hooked up to every machine known to man in that area, blood was taken, and two doctors were assigned to me. I was not awake when Tom arrived as I had within the previous hour passed out cold. Almost immediately the doctors intubated me with a breathing tube. My body had begun to shut down – my liver, kidneys, and blood pressure. It took a few hours for the doctors to determine exactly what was causing this situation, concluding for sure it was some kind of bacterial infection, but they did not immediately know what type. As it turned out I had sepsis. Sepsis can kill a healthy person very quickly; never mind me with a severely weakened immune system. When Tom arrived at my ICU room the doctors told him that all they knew at the moment was that I had a "gram rod negative bacterial infection," but what kind, and how I got it, they did not know. They informed Tom immediately as well that they had only two hours to figure out exactly what I had or I would die.

"Does Stacey have a living will?" the doctors asked Tom.

Tom was shattered by this question but said, "Yes, she does."

"Get it" was the reply.

As Tom set about calling my personal attorney, who is a most excellent friend to me, Tom and he spoke about the contents of the living will and where it was located. To this day Tom barely remembers anything in detail that happened in those few hours or much of the ongoing conversations. He was in severe shock.

A team of doctors from Brigham and Women's Hospital as well as Mass General were furiously working to figure out which antibiotic to give me. The right one would save my life; the wrong one would not. The doctors indicated to Tom that while they were not certain exactly which infection I had, they had an idea it was a nasty *E. coli* and that with the way I was declining they had no choice but to guess on one of three possible medications and hope it was correct. Brigham's at this exact time did not have in house the specific antibiotic that they wanted to treat me with, so they needed to secure the IV bags from Mass General. The doctors, thank God, obviously guessed correctly.

I later learned that my *E. coli* infection had resulted from several slowly developing and unrecognized issues, which had been going on inside me for several long weeks. Their conclusion was that I was suffering serious stress as a result of trying to work again. Internal stress mostly, but this stress in turn caused my internal flora (or good intestinal gut bacteria) to be overwhelmed with bad intestinal bacteria. As this grew it took over my intestinal area, causing my gallbladder to become infected, which in turn sent an infection throughout my body up and into my port area. By the time of July Fourth, it was like a bomb going off in my body, resulting in my fever of 103.5°, the final warning my body was giving me. Sepsis had definitely set in. I did not have a lot of time left once this happened and getting into the hospital to be correctly diagnosed was most imperative. Tom saved my life by calling Christina to be with me. If he had not done this, I most definitely would have died that day at home.

Thankfully, for myself, I was on a breathing machine for a couple of days and did not wake up at all. When I did, I can recall seeing two young female doctors with me, carrying back and forth small IV bags on and off the pole next to me. When my nurse saw that I was awake, she raced immediately out into the hall, saying as she left, "Your husband is just outside, I will get him!"

Flying into my room in less than a few seconds, Tom sat on my left side. He took my hands, came in close to my face, and looked deep into my eyes. *"Welcome back, beautiful,"* he said. I had seen Tom stare into my eyes before with deep feeling, but this time, I could not take my eyes off of his. It was as if Tom could see down deep into my soul. His eyes were penetrating me with a force of will and love such as I had never seen. I knew my husband loved me. But I never knew *how much* until that exact moment. I will remember this feeling until my last day on Earth.

In looking at Tom I felt like I was in a dream. A really beautiful dream, until I noticed something felt odd and I looked down at myself after a few minutes and realized then that I was wearing a diaper. I could not help it, I felt embarrassed by this, and so I whispered, "I am wearing a diaper, Tom," and he smiled back at me, not taking his eyes off mine, and said, "I know, love, it's okay ... you've been very sick."

At that moment too I noticed again the young female doctors in my room. They each appeared to be around twenty years old and I asked Tom who they were because they looked like cheerleaders to me, and he told me that they were the doctors who had been taking care of me. *Wow,* I thought to myself, *how incredible this all was. The doctors barely looked old enough to be out of college.* Looking back at Tom, he was just smiling and staring at me. I had no idea at all, nor did Tom tell me for a very long time, just how close I had come to dying. He simply did not tell me nor did the doctors.

I fell back to sleep after visiting with Tom for a little longer and I stayed asleep for many long hours. I slept for days actually, only waking here and there. By far, this hospital stay, which was again over three full weeks, was the most difficult I have ever experienced. I went through constant tests, MRIs, x-rays, CT scans, over and over tests, more tests, more blood work, etc. I was exhausted every time I woke up. My arms were horribly black and blue, each of them, from all of the different IVs, blood draws, etc. Often during the middle of the night, I would awaken to see a nurse assistant sitting in the chair next to me, just waiting to be near for when I woke up. While I had no idea for several months after discharge how close to death I had been, what I could see was that this hospital stay had been a very difficult one for everyone in my family. Stress and deep sadness were in everyone's eyes when I awoke to see one of my brothers with me, or all of them together sitting in my room. While they were always smiling at me and encouraging that I not be worried about needing to fall back to sleep, I could hear in my mind the echo of the look I saw briefly in their faces. They were worried, each of them, deeply. I could see this with Tom too when Tom was there, which was almost always. A very close call indeed this was. But again, by the hand of God, I was pulled through. Sepsis kills most people who contract it because it attacks fast and hard and normally by the time the hospital figures out what caused it, the patient has gone too far into decline.

The reality was that my recovery from having sepsis was much more difficult than the recovery from my stem cell transplant. I was seventy pounds heavier from body fluid resulting from the insult and assault on my lymphatic and nervous system. My lymphatic system was unable to easily release the extreme fluid load. I could barely walk; in fact at first, I could not walk. I could not lift myself up any type of incline step, not even a very small sidewalk step or curb. It was awful. It was hot and humid this summer and the heat itself would add to my discomfort. But I had Tom, Christina, and Jeff, and they never left my side for long, taking turns to see that I was never alone. I needed help up and down all the stairs at home. Tom literally had to lift me up from underneath my arms to help me climb the stairs to bed, back down again at night to use the bathroom, and then down again another set of steps into the family room during the day. I was unable to write legibly for months. I could not remember my own phone number for weeks, nor my address and other simple daily facts. It was in many ways as if I was recovering from having suffered a stroke.

When Tom and Christina needed to head out for a family event one day several weeks after I got back home, Jeffrey stayed with me this entire day, his only day off from work that week. He rested in the chair next to me for over ten hours. It was a very hot August day outside and even though the backyard pool was open, Jeff never left me alone. He snoozed, got me drinks and food, and when I wanted to go outside for a breath of air, he would help me down the slight step from the house onto the ground and back up again. Not once, ever, did Jeffrey look at me with eyes that spoke of any frustration or desire to be anywhere else. Total acceptance and unconditional love was the way he looked at me whenever he came over to see if I needed anything. *How blessed am I,* I can remember thinking, when Jeff came over to my side mid-afternoon with his beautiful eyes alive with love and concern, asking if I was okay and did I need anything at all. Always for me, it is about the eyes. "The mirror to one's soul" is the saying, is it not? I can attest to that completely. No one can hide any lies when their eyes are so close to yours.

So it was as well with Christina. One morning as she was helping me down the family room stairs, my legs – so heavy and clumsy with fluid – gave out completely, and I fell right on top of her. Somehow, Christina got up and picked me up fully without hurting me or herself, her eyes full of compassion and concern that I not have gotten hurt. My heart filled with such love for her. Today my inner being still radiates with warmth whenever I remember how kind her eyes were at this exact moment. And while I felt so loved and cared for by my family, I was tired and very weary from being ill. The long days were hard for me and I was oftentimes dazed, feeling completely diluted in my abilities. I had not experienced for a long while any angelic visits such as before, but one night after an especially dispiriting week I had an amazing vision/dream. Vividly, I can recall becoming aware of sitting on my farmhouse kitchen floor. Morning light came in through the windows. I was sitting cross-legged and as I turned to look up, I could see the hazy outline of someone with me, but I could not tell who. Then very gently my cat Bailey, who had died years before, was handed down for me to hold. It was as though he was poured into my arms, and when I felt him fully, I pulled him close to me – hugging him tightly, as tight as I could. I was able to smell his special scent and feel his fur and I could hear him purring, his gentle loving purr that was always *his* special sound. I knew while I was holding Bailey that I was having a dream-vision that on an inner dimensional level was totally real, and as such was a special gift. So I concentrated hard to make this experience last, and it did last for what seemed several long minutes. How I loved holding Bailey, knowing and feeling deep in my heart that he loved me still, and that our special bond existed beyond the veil of time, forever. Suddenly, I awoke and for several minutes I could still feel Bailey with me in spirit, and I knew then that I would see him again someday. He was waiting for me someplace special. I knew this deep in my soul. How I cherished that experience. It helped me to heal a deep wound that had been with me for such a long time. Bailey had gone missing long year's prior and never returned home again. His loss and not knowing what happened to him, where he went and how he died, caused me deep sorrow. I never stopped thinking of him, praying one day to know the truth, and now I did. Bailey was in heaven and he and I will be together again someday.

A few months later after this amazing vision/dream of Bailey, Tom and I were up at the lake house for a weekend visit, our first since my being home from the hospital. Jeffrey was with us that Sunday afternoon. Late in the day there had been a brief rain shower. As I was sitting outside on our deck, Jeffrey suddenly came running up the long path from where he had been fishing with Tom. He was yelling for me to look up at the sky, "**There is an incredible rainbow overhead, Stacey, look!!**" As I turned around and looked up I saw that the rainbow arch was directly positioned over the house with us right smack in the middle. The rainbow colors were amazingly crisp, clear, and beautiful. With a beaming smile I could see Jeff was conveying to me that he saw this rainbow as a "sign" somehow – a gift that I would be well again soon. As Jeffrey went back to the water, minutes later another rainbow appeared. Jeff again shouted to me excitedly to look up again. When I saw this double rainbow, the feeling of joy that radiated through my body was intense, and as I looked down again at Jeffrey smiling up at me, in that moment, I felt a special connection to him that deepened my faith that I was exactly in my life where God wanted me to be and all would be well.

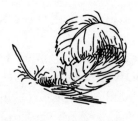

CHAPTER 9

Releasing the Past

I<small>F</small> G<small>OD HAD ANY PURPOSE FOR ME IN HAVING BECOME SO ILL, FOR</small> so long, I believe one of the reasons may have been for me to have experienced the love and care from my family as I did: experiences that were never a part of my life when I was single and living a busy businesswoman's life. I have inside me indelible memories of pure unconditional love for me, by my stepchildren and my husband. And as terrible as my illness and setbacks have been, I am so grateful for each moment that they shared themselves with me like this, allowing the truth of their feelings for me to be seen, so that my soul, where hidden injury had lived for far too long, not yet touched by anything else in my life, had a chance to be nurtured in this way. *My family healed me deeply.* And I love them beyond words because of it. Maybe this is one of the mystical truths as to the reason "why" I did get cancer. Maybe herein lays the "gift" that my soul most needed.

Once the worst of the water retention was behind me, my weight went right back down to a very low level. It was hard for me to look at myself in the mirror as I did not recognize the frail woman in front of me. So I followed one nurse's advice. She had said simply, "Do not look at you, Stacey. Give your body time to heal," she instructed, "do not focus on how you look. Your beauty will come back during the bloom phase." I looked forward to that ... "the bloom phase," when a transplant patient's body begins to fully heal and they regain their prior visage, sometimes healthier if they had been ill for a long time before diagnosis.

The second year of recovery was a bit easier. I was able to go to the grocery store and handle the bags coming back into the house. In general, I was feeling better and began trying once again to do more work, not realizing just yet that I would never be able to return to my prior capacity, as I was before my illness. But, I tried, and I held out hope, as did my partners. But during 2011, whenever I suffered stress, I got ill, and the cycle of upset did not abate. My partners and employees were in a sense waiting for me to return, to pick up where I had left off, and while I tried and worked emails to stay connected, I would never again return to the role of CEO/President in any true full-time capacity.

The economy during my stem cell transplant and initial recovery was most difficult and the company unexpectedly lost many long-standing customers to both private label selections and competitor items. In fact, during the first few days of my hospital stay for the transplant, we had lost one more very solid customer that I personally handled that had over 1,000 stores to which we had sold our items for over fourteen years. This was on the heels of losing three large national chains with over 3,000 stores combined the previous twelve months, a terrible blow to the company that had nothing to do with our products' quality or our sales level and everything to do with each supermarket chain's private label goals and/or that of a competitor. I can recall praying upon hearing the news of the last chain loss, "Dear God, please do not tell me I have come here into this hospital to have my life saved, only to watch my company die." I was heartbroken at what was occurring, but too far gone into my own body's decline to think more on it. But in the back of my mind, I could hear the message, *it will not die, but it will look different later on. And it is not just for you to save.*

Despite the unfortunate change in the dynamics of the company's sales, I could not jump back into my old position and this began to cause me terrible pain by early 2012. I was struggling with deep feelings of intense sadness, guilt, and failure. I kept thinking that if I had not become sick, maybe I would have been able to blunt the loss of several chains. I could not stop thinking of my earlier days, my successes, how I handled difficult day-to-day business issues, and the good results I could affect with my personal touch. I would never be that person again, never again ... and this knowing caused me at times terrible, body-racking pain. With my spiritual books in hand and Tom by my side, I could not stop the emotional storms from happening and they began to happen often. I would feel deep despair for days at a time. Inconsolable crying occurred – something I just never did, crying for many hours and days. I was in deep despair because I could not "do" what I used to be able to do to protect and help my company, and I felt so much guilt. Despite my strong spiritual belief that all would be well, this road was foreign and I was so afraid that innocent people inside the company would lose their jobs and friends of the company would be irreparably hurt.

As this pain continued, it became clear to me by the

early spring of 2012 that I would need counseling to help me through these episodes. I was referred to a wonderful therapist at the Survivorship Clinic at Dana Farber and began visits immediately. By my third session with my therapist, she helped me to accept what was no longer to be my life, and to understand that what I was experiencing was in essence true "grieving." I was *grieving* the loss of who I had been as a person before my cancer and that in many ways, that person had died ... and a new Stacey had been born. I knew that of course was true physically, but never did I put together for myself that the pain I was experiencing was not in reality "guilt," because I was in fact not guilty of having done anything wrong. I was, though, "grieving." That knowing hit me directly in the heart as being right, and I could feel myself relax in my therapist's presence. Yes, of course! I am grieving ... *how could I not be?* And in a few more short weeks of follow-up, I had the tools I needed to process these feelings without undue emotional upset. What I was going through was perfectly normal and all I needed was more time to accept who I was no longer going to be in my new life.

After realizing what I was actually experiencing, and with Tom's help, I determined that I would need to resign as the company's CEO/President. Before I did that, though, I needed to prepare my business partners for this reality. I took steps to do so, and as often as I could, but it was not easy. The company was still in distress and it seemed, I was always needed to attend to some issue or item that if left unattended would/could cycle into wholesale disaster for the company. The company needed a leader. It needed someone to be watching out for its interests as I always had done. My founding partner had all he could do to keep up with his side of the business, which is the plant operation. However, there were other partners/shareholders too and whether they wanted to help out the company or not, I could no longer wait for them to act directly on behalf of the company. I needed for my own health and well-being to resign. So in April 2012, I tendered my resignation as CEO/President of the company that I founded some twenty-seven years earlier. A few short months later a deep healing did began to take place for me. My immune system showed improvement and in my mind I felt calmness. I began to be able to see the company more objectively, although not perfectly always ... but better than before. It was clear to me that it was up to the other company partners to determine going forward how best to work without me, even though the daily office affairs still needed tender guidance from me.

As the summer approached its end, it was, I unfortunately discovered, absolutely impossible to cut myself off completely from ongoing management needs, that only I knew best how to handle. Tom felt I was retarding the company's acceptance of my inability to come back, and maybe that was to a high degree true. But I was still a major shareholder and allowing problems to snowball into crisis because young new office staff had no clue how to fix things seemed irresponsible. To me, it was like leaving a soldier out on the battlefield while he or she was bleeding. I could not do that ... and so for a long time, I continued to suffer energy loss that my body needed for further healing, by way of allowing into my day stressful hours and revolving stressful demands. I turned each morning to prayer, and for help in finding clues as to why again, a chronic condition within the company could not resolve itself.

As I reached for my spiritual books for comfort and

guidance, time and again I got many answers. For example, I knew that in the big picture, God has steered my life onto an exit ramp, and that I needed to stay on this new road I was traveling. I call it "the scenic route" of my life, and I needed to consciously remember that, and remain on it, enjoying the view out the window, and the slower speed. It was a deep knowing within me that if I tried to figure out a way how to get back up and onto the freeway of my prior life in business, it will lead to a fatality. Somehow, some way my life will end. And I would not do that, not ever. I owe too much to the people who have healed me, my family, my doctors and my nurses, my insurance company that took such good care of me and my bills, and my loyal friends and neighbors who have enriched my life so much. *No, I am never going back up there ever again.* Accepting this fact inside my inner soul was a struggle because I love my company, our employees, and my partner, who is a talented man. So, for a long time, I straddled, while trying to find a way to do just enough, not too much, but to be available for those who still needed me. The company had essentially been and still was … too much "me" so breaking away from this kind of umbilical cord tie was not easy, but for my future health and mental stability, it turned into a must.

How to do that? How to make that break? This was the most difficult part of my healing. I relied constantly on my books, especially those from White Eagle. Always soothing, always perfect were the messages for the moment, and for the situation. But no matter those words, it was still incumbent upon me to take the necessary actions I knew finally would lead me to my future.

In writing these words now, I have asked myself how can I share or offer an example of the beauty and enrichment these wonderful works have provided me for all these past years. The answer comes very quickly. *Select any page that comes to mind.* And that page for me, right at this moment, is page 51 in White Eagle's *Heal Thyself.* What a great title, *Heal Thyself,* meaning to each of us that on many levels we have it within our control and God-authorized power to heal ourselves. We just have to try.

Here are White Eagle's words:

> Develop from the heart, meditate on love, live love, absorb love, give love, and your soul will become alight. The divine magic will rest in your hands enabling you to heal the sick, to comfort the bereaved, to bless the sorrowful, to beautify everything you touch, and to bring peace and happiness to the life of man.

That has been my heart's mission. I want to achieve a peaceful life, but in reaching for that new life, I want to offer love to those remaining behind and without me. The people in my life that I have been able to speak to about this fully and without reservation and who I knew would not judge me were my youngest brother Michael and my wonderful brothers Brian and Tim. I am able to call each of them at any time and share with them my deepest fears and my inner conflict. Each of them supported me in every way to trust that I had given my company "**everything**" and that I had to slowly, and with grace ... "LET GO."

A Soft Landing. Arrival into a beautiful new reality whereby one can release oneself from a turbulent life that no longer should be lived-- trusting and knowing that your greatest good and the good of others is protected and in the hands of God. Right action is called forth in all ways of being, thinking, and acting. This spiritual "truth" is supported here also in White Eagle's words one paragraph earlier:

> Every time you give way to passion and anger you dissipate the holy fire; every time emotions are controlled and transmuted to the warmth of love, you build the light into your vehicles [meaning your soul and body] ... You are using the divine fire to illumine your own soul, to beautify the world about you and to glorify God.

To glorify God is a form of (feeling) prayer and develops within the ability to sense the boundaries of what is right action and what is wrong action in trying to understand any difficult situation. To learn to walk in peace and to be able to release things which a person no longer is, but to do that completely and with integrity, one benefits greatly thinking in terms of glorifying God. It becomes like an inner compass. God IS and God's work is perfect however events turn out. If I am troubled, a transformation immediately happens inside my mind whenever I pray or do my spiritual readings. Suddenly, I know what it is exactly that I need to do for my life. Like lightning the needed steps come into my mind, and I can surrender again and trust that "yes," all is well and as it should be.

Often it is true for many people who have been critically sick, and whose lives have been saved by the wonderful medicines available today, that immediately following recovery, one wants so much to enter a new chapter in life. Charity work may become an obsessive need for many, while others are left just trying to find ways to say "thank you," with heartfelt gratitude, for the wonderful medicines, and for the doctors and nurses who saved their lives. This is especially true for people who are in their younger years or who are middle aged.

So many years still to live!

For myself, one realization that I gained during recovery is that prior to being severely ill, I never really paid a lot of attention to other people who passed me by every day. I was living a whirlwind of hours here and there, everywhere. When at the grocery store, I never paid any mind to others in the aisles shopping or to the cashier who may have been having a horrible day. No, it was always, "get in, get out, I've got a lot to do ... do you mind moving it along, people." I was never rude, but I was always in a rush. Not anymore. Not today. I discovered that it was important to me, in the early days of being able once again to go grocery shopping, that I notice others, all around me, who were very often themselves in a physical recovery of some kind. So I paid attention, and I noticed things I never saw before. For example, I began to go to my local Market Basket at 7:15 AM, to shop, just after they opened. It was always very quiet inside, but still there was a good handful of people, who like me, appeared to be unwell or disabled. Many were seniors and others who just looked like they needed a lot more time to walk the store aisles without being rushed. *Who knew this world existed?* I asked myself after a few trips. Wow, how out of touch was I. It began to matter to me, if I could reach up to grab a box of pasta, when someone near me needed help. I became more alert, and watched what was happening around me, and with the other shoppers. I often was moving quite slowly myself, and those who were shopping near me could see that, and very often one of them would smile at me ... *that knowing smile* that said gently, "hang in there ... you're doing great." *And I was!* I was shopping for my family, after not having been able to for so long. A victory to be proud of and I was proud! I showed that pride and happiness by smiling at the cashiers even though I was still masked. But even masked they could see I was smiling and they almost always smiled back.

I needed to take my time out to the car each trip, and in the unpacking of the car, and in so doing I would see birds flying all around and feel the soft breeze, little things I never noticed before. Our Market Basket always has the nicest flowers and potted plants outside their store during the spring and summer, and I took the time to really look at them, appreciating the store's efforts in their presentation and enjoying them being there every day that I went shopping. Because it was so early in the day, the feeling to the air was at times almost silky, and I came to see these plants and flowers as greeting me: "Good morning, Stacey, welcome!"

And I did feel welcomed in this store. If I wanted a special iced tea drink made from green tea, they ordered it for me. If I wanted a special butter from Ireland, they ordered it. It was like being cared for on a different level from people I barely knew. But I was a customer, and they cared that I got what it was that I wanted. And just this small effort made me feel that I was on my way back from having been brought so low.

Standing tall and holding poise throughout my terrible physical fragility, after having been so vital and vibrant in my earlier life, was essential to me as a human being. Achieving this poise was always aided intensely by my spiritual books and prayers.

Other parts of White Eagle's words I read and reread

for inspiration and fulfillment daily were many. One such passage that I rely on often reads:

> When you concentrate upon negative things you give them life, but if you cease to think about them you withdraw life from them and they gradually die. People say, "Oh, but we do not want to turn our backs on reality, we must face it." But, my children, reality is light; reality is all that is positive, good, pure and true. It is what you call evil that is unreal. Always concentrate on goodness, beauty and love.

Further down it continues:

> There is always something beautiful to be found. Look for it: Concentrate on it. This positive loving attitude towards life and people helps you to perceive their divine essence, to put into operation the divine magic which heals. ... The purpose of man's life is that he shall grow towards consciousness of his own God-qualities, and the way to do this is for him continually to rise in thought to the spheres of light, continually to open himself to the constructive forces and creative power of God.

As I walk now on my new path, and towards my new life, and as I look forward to the future I know that is near, I am refreshed each time when I read these words and works. These books that offer such serenity and comfort never grow old; no matter how many times I may read from the same book, the same words, and feel again their meaning, sometimes they affect me as if I am reading them again for the very first time. It is helpful to think and remember that all of us are like young children, learning and growing on this road home to God consciousness. But I am stronger, I am surer, I am more awake and aware that I am heading where I am meant to be. That is the source of my greatest comfort today.

White Eagle offers this thought too:

> The demands of modern life seem so urgent that you forget the grave importance and need of inner communion, the breaking of the bread of life. This, together with loving service in the world, will build into your being particles of light, transmuting the darkness and which will overcome the destructive forces which play around and within you. This is the secret of the transmutation of the dark, dull, heavy metals of gross matter into the pure gold of spirit.

Or in other words: *Alchemy*. When I was younger I was fascinated by the idea of alchemy, the theory that base metals could be turned into gold. I never found any scientific evidence that such could be achieved, but I certainly thought *maybe*. Now I realize that what I was actually searching for was the magic that is found only in the spiritual transmutation of turning darkness and fear into the peace, love, and calmness that comes from finding God within. This is true alchemy, and within reach of every person who truly desires to transform himself or herself, leaving behind their individual fears, and "choosing" to live in peace and harmony.

I have learned that life never has to be as difficult as

we make it to be. I believe totally in the basic goodness of most everyone, although for sure, there are truly evil people in this world. But they in their evilness are often sick and misguided. I pray for them, and hope in some small way, this helps. I used to think maybe I could find a way to help these people directly, and then I realized that is not the road God wants me on. So I have abandoned any feelings of "trying to save the world." God will save the world, and it will happen when he decides. But in the meantime, I can live a wonderful happy life with Tom and the kids, and I do not need to feel responsible to fix happenings outside of my control and personal power. I have enough to contend with staying on the path of stronger health, daily living with joy in simple things like preparing a delicious meal and in being with my animals that are so much a part of my daily life, and of course loving Tom.

Finding true inner peace is essential. Prayer leads me back to that every time. The more often I pray the quicker I can be rebalanced if for any reason something throws me off. It is my hope that anyone who is reading my words gives prayer a try, and if you do pray now already, I hope that some of the words I have shared strengthen your resolve to remain on the path you know will keep you sound, whole, and connected to God.

Growth as a soul in this world of misty shadows and grey edges can be very harsh and cold. It is easy to become despondent, depressed, and lonely. Afraid ... *that everyone and everything is against you.* Of course, if you are alone and without God inside you, you can be almost defenseless and you will suffer, suffering sometimes terribly, before you are ready to secure for yourself true peace inside your soul. But just like the story of the Prodigal Son, when you are ready to return home, God is there waiting for you with open arms. *How I love that story.* It means no matter how far away from God any of us may have traveled, no matter how difficult our lessons, no matter how deep in pain we may be, no matter the pain we may have caused others, when we have had enough and we want to return "home" where we will feel nurtured, safe, and loved, all we need to do is to turn our hearts and eyes towards God, and there He instantly IS!

As White Eagle wrote in *Heal Thyself*:

> One of the lessons which the candidate [who we all are] on the path to spiritual illuminations has to learn is that nothing can really touch or hurt him. The natural physical instinct is to fear, but the spirit of truth within you has to bring through into full consciousness the knowledge that no harm can touch the real you. Encourage this thought until it is always with you. Nothing can harm you and there is nothing to fear except fear. If you have full confidence in God the white light will flow through your being and all darkness will be eliminated. Live quietly, tranquilly in God's love. Every life which is of God is crowned by love, which is a supreme and perfect happiness.

A Soft Landing ... how sweet is this feeling. Knowing that no matter how much pain or how far away from God we may have traveled, we can always come back home and rest within Him.

It does not matter how big your home is, how many things you may own, or how much money you have in the bank. God will provide, of that you can be assured. Perfectly and in "His" way, you will never be cold, afraid, hungry, or alone. But, first you must allow Him in.

Throughout much of my life I have known this truth, but I have forgotten. It has been for me tippy-toe steps. I was just so distracted for so many years of my life. But today I am free from that and my life is anew. Every morning when I wake up, I am filled with gratitude and joy. The echoing sounds of the lake and the birds, and the soft early morning light coming in through my front windows, make me so happy. I am safe. I am home. I am healthy in mind, spirit, and heart, living daily with the knowledge that it can remain this way forever.

Words to hold close to your heart

> Every soul seems to suffer; but if you can see that suffering in its right perspective you will see that it brings a rebirth. Through limitation and suffering the soul emerges into the divine life and light, just as the insect emerges from the chrysalis stage into a beautiful winged creature in the sunlight.
>
> White Eagle – *Heal Thyself*

> He that dwelleth in the secret place of the most High shall abide under the shadow of the Almighty ... He shall cover thee with his **FEATHERS**, and under his wings shall thou trust.
>
> Psalms 91:1, 4

> God's creation dwells in Love ... Of this we may be sure that thoughts winged with peace and

love breathe a silent benediction over all the earth, cooperate with the divine power and brood unconsciously over the work of His hand ... Thus founded upon the rock of Christ, when storm and tempest beat against this sure foundation, you, safely sheltered in the strong tower of hope, faith and Love, are God's nestlings: and He will hide you in His **FEATHERS** till the storm has passed. Into His haven of Soul there enters no element of earth to cast out angels, to silence the right intuition which guides you safely home.

Mary Baker Eddy
"Haven of the Soul," *Miscellaneous Writings 1883–1896*, p. 152.

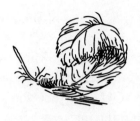

CHAPTER 10

Love Heals All

HAVE OFTEN BEEN ASKED BY THE FEW WITH WHOM I HAVE SHARED my personal story why I have had these incredible experiences and not someone else – even if they with all their hearts believe in God. I know from having read many spiritual writings that it is not uncommon for God to speak directly to any individual who is receptive in his or her senses. He or she may not be aware of God's voice just yet. Many religions promise peace, serenity, love, and security in coming to know God intimately. And most religions believe that God is somewhere, doing amazing things. But if your goal is to personally connect with God, and to have him be a part of your daily life and a voice within your soul, while I am not an expert, I hope I can make certain recommendations that will help you find a way to communicate with and keep a connection with God.

I believe firmly in a few basic Universal Truths. Universal Truths just **are**, no matter one's color, ethnic background, religion or no religion, or where one lives in the world. My mom has a saying that is one of the highest truths in life: "You take YOU wherever you GO." And this statement, which I heard so often while growing up, helped shape my basic character, and my self-awareness. Knowing that YOU are responsible for YOU, and that you cannot escape yourself, no matter what or no matter where you go, immediately places personal responsibility onto yourself for everything: how you perceive life, your relationships, everything. No matter how far you run away from something, one day you will turn around and see ... **"THERE YOU ARE."**

If you maintain any level of self-consciousness and self-awareness in this life, you will always know your own personal truth. And part of this universal truth is that there is no place to hide, except in your own mind, where maybe you set up a kabuki theatre in which you use masks to hide from yourself. But as time passes, life has a way of uncovering one's dark secrets, lies, and evil. **God is GOOD.** We are his creation and every person, no matter who, has a part of God within him or her. You can ignore this truth, blaspheme His name and commit horrible acts against yourself and others, but you are going nowhere in the end. God IS. And He will be there waiting for you on your final day, and that is a solid truth I believe with all my heart and soul.

How to connect with God? Try starting by saying the Lord's Prayer often. Say it with feeling, reverence, and true desire and God will awaken inside your soul. He will begin to speak in a voice not unlike your own inner conscious mind, but it will have a different ring or tone to it. Listen for this and continue to pray. I have found that I can amplify my own connection with God by obeying the words and advice that I hear. If I am guided to not drive to the store at a particular moment, I simply do not. If I am prompted to make a phone call to a friend, I do. Normally, I find there is always good reason for that call to have been made. If I see a stray or injured animal, I stop and do all that I can to aid that small living being. That is how God and His ways are strengthened and how they grow.

Miracles come from God, but many small daily miracles can occur when inner guidance is obeyed and intuitions are respected and followed. The results are often that difficult situations improve. Crisis is calmed. Health worries are eased and pain is often either reduced or eliminated. Always, though, *know that God has the final say*. Asking for something that you want does not in fact mean you will get it. However, in the asking, trust how your life unfolds, as you begin to work with awareness that God resides within you. It is truly uncanny how in the end, your best interests are always served in exactly the right way. This for me was also a great lesson. Relaxing and trusting that if I stopped pushing, my good result desired would arrive. It just might not look exactly as I had hoped or thought it would, but when it arrived, always, once I realized that it was here – it was better than what I had dreamt or hoped it would be.

Metaphysics tells us that positive thinking is capable of producing positive reality as well. Thoughts are real. You can do much healing for yourself and others by simply reversing your tendency towards negative thinking by saying "cancel that," and reintroducing your true intention, especially if your intentions are good. The true intentions behind your words and thoughts are real and have real consequences. If you act with good will, you do put forth the energy of healing to those around you, no matter the circumstances. Believe in good, and good will arrive in your life.

One of the most important things I can recommend is to

LOVE. Love yourself. Love your family (even if you do not like some of them). LOVE is the most potent force on earth. God is Love and Love heals all. Pure unconditional love is a universal gift available to every person, because LOVE IS everywhere. Believing that you deserve love in your life means you are on the way to having love be a part of your everyday experience. It can be. So shall it be. Tap into this knowing and your life will bloom and you will feel joy.

Every day, all around us people are suffering. Small animals are suffering acts of unimaginable cruelty. You yourself may be suffering. You may have been the cause of intense suffering for someone else. The very best way to heal this reality is to become a light in someone else's life, and watch magic happen in yours. If every person alive and on Earth today contributed something of themselves to just one person, or in the helping of a small creature, suffering would slowly end. It simply would. And while this truth simply IS true, you do not have to wait for a grand gesture to get started. You do not have to approach it by trying to save the world. Baby steps are all that is needed. The very act of helping someone in pain or difficulty or by way of helping a small injured animal reaffirms your own innocence within your soul and awakens a compassion which is most beautiful.

Small animals are here on earth to be our companions. The painful things people do to them are very hard to witness, and often this happens because the animal is seen as an object without feeling or sensation. Indifference towards small animals is rampant in the world. When someone thoughtlessly abandons or disregards an animal, this kind of action cycles and evolves. You can help end that in a small but significant way.

Don't.

Don't disregard an innocent animal needing your help or one that comes into your field of awareness. Every time an injured or hungry animal comes into your range of sight, this is a special gift of sorts for you. If you do not have the resources or ability to care for this animal, most veterinarians will accept a stray dog or cat and in turn find a shelter for them. If you have an animal shelter nearby, please take the animal there. Just don't leave it, especially if it is a stray, to be further starved and neglected. There is no greater immediate reward for a soul seeking nurturing and spiritual growth than helping a small living creature that on its own cannot repair its situation. Help, be a light for that which you see, without delay. Don't be too busy, too broke, or too disinterested. It takes so little to do so much good. Allow yourself to embrace your humanity through feelings of inner compassion. Compassion is not pity. Pity is in actuality a form of judgment whereby you feel you are superior to an inferior situation you are witnessing. Pity is not pretty, nor does it offer love. Compassion is the essential glue which binds all living beings to each other and is the essence of true purity and real love. Compassion awakened will heal instantly that which you may have been unable to find remedy for. Trust that in life there is no deeper mystery to be solved or puzzle to be figured out than to discover completely that compassion simply is God in motion from one living being to another.

You can extend this love once discovered towards a neighbor who may need a hand in small chores or physical assistance. Begin to "see" your own innocence by recognizing in others their innocence, as well the innocence that exists within all other living beings. In so doing, your life will be saved no matter what your past may have been. It matters not whether you personally enjoy the neighbor or the person you are helping. Just help. Be of good heart in any way that you can.

Start in your own home, your neighborhood, your town, wherever you feel called to help. Helping just one person with homecare or grocery shopping, or aiding a stray hungry animal is an act of love that will resonate all around you, inside you, inside the person or being you are helping. *Healing will happen.* Suddenly, you are not so tired anymore. Your desperation and/or your depression eases. Laughter happens more easily and, in general, your sleep is much deeper. Caring for someone, anyone, or any small helpless creature is a healing force like no other. If prayer does not feel right for you at this time, then care for someone other than yourself, and you will be on the road to true healing in many ways.

In my life today, one of the best living examples I know of someone who lives this truth is my brother Brian. He and a few of his very close friends, separately and together, live and walk their faith every day. They leave groceries on the front doorstep of families they know have a real need. They do this all year, not just at Christmas time. No acknowledgment note is left of who did this, they just DO! Children and teenagers in need of special help receive it by way of anonymous monies for college or special education by a couple of Brian's close friends. Youths at risk are given foster care or oversight care by one of them. They watch, they listen individually, and as a group, and as a caring community aid those around them who are known to be in real need, without any consideration or expectation of recognition or honor. I admire Brian and his friends deeply for this and whenever Brian is near me I can see inside him a shining bright light. Truly, he is a man who walks a godly life even while he will be the first to tell you, he is not a perfect human being. No one is, but he is in my eyes very close to one. And Brian is one of the happiest men I know. He laughs with great ease, he jokes with everyone, he opens his home to friends and family without reservation and when he is near you he is "present"; he is awake and aware. Most important in my admiration of how Brian lives his life today is that he is someone who suffered severe physical challenges and multiple surgeries as a young child. His soul was softened by these experiences I am sure, and instead of being a hard and resentful man, Brian is full of gratitude in all that he has, his wife, his family, and his friends.

The Universal Truth "love thy neighbor" is an ancient proverb largely ignored by (us) humans. This is such a simple and basic Truth and not a difficult one at all to make a reality. If every human being cared for the well-being of just one other person, the Earth would be slowly trans-formed. It is a mathematical certainty.

God has sent many prophets and messengers to provide guidance to humans: Abraham, Moses, Jesus, Mohammed, Buddha, and others. And despite the huge financial resources dedicated to churches, mosques, temples, and sanctuaries, suffering still exists everywhere. It still is too much a part of the collective human condition.

Baby steps ...

It is my deepest hope that if my words inspire and moti-vate you, that you trust that in the act of helping just one other person – you begin the ways of true healing for all.

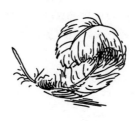

Epilogue

A S I NEARED THE END OF THIS WRITING, MY FIRST INSPIRA-
tional book, the universe handed me an unexpected
surprise. While at a follow-up visit with my oncol-
ogist, during month three of year three in recovery – February 2013 – I received good news. My kidneys, which had
been so negatively affected by all of the medications, treatments, and prior failures due to sepsis, were now showing
recovery. The test results that day showed NORMAL readings. I had been told during the past two years not to really
expect that my kidneys would return to normal levels. So,
I had accepted that they may always be a little "hot" or
slightly abnormal. What a wonderful and unexpected gift.

But not more than one week later, I received an email
from Dr. Antin that my PCR results were just in and that
they were slightly elevated, and that he wanted to begin
as a response a new chemotherapy medication to reverse
this. I asked "What does this mean in lay terms"? My
doctor replied that the "Philadelphia Chromosome, which
is the marker for CML (leukemia) was now present again

and slightly elevated." In other words, I was no longer in a "cured" state. However, my doctor added, not to fear, the medication would knock it back down into remission.

Tom was with me when I read this email and he immediately broke down. Never have I seen him so demoralized and heartbroken. Tom's reaction was much more intense than the worst moments for us in the early months of my diagnosis and transplant.

"WHY"?? I asked myself, "WHY is this happening now?" I felt almost nothing about this new result and was to be honest a little surprised. "WHY am I not more upset?"

I emailed back and forth with my doctor to seek answers because Tom was spiraling again into a very dark place emotionally. Dr. Antin responded with calmness that it is just not unusual for the cancer to reawaken. But still, even if this is a common enough relapse, Tom and I never thought this could ever re-occur for me. How could it? I was cured by my transplant, wasn't I??

Within a day, after Tom had a chance to calm a bit, we went away for short trip of skiing, staying at one of our favorite hotels near home. During that time I had a chance to pray and consider things. The answer that came to me over and over was to "dis-create" this event. I'd never had this type of thought before. But, I decided as a result not to announce immediately to my family that leukemia had returned. I felt that I needed to accept that for whatever reason, I was faced again with another chance to exercise my faith and heal myself totally. When Tom returned from skiing, refreshed and relaxed we spoke about the reappearance of the cancer and how to consider it. I discussed with Tom that I was intuitively sensing that I needed to "dis-create" my leukemia by giving its arrival (however slight) zero power over us and our daily life. We needed to acknowledge it, treat it with the medication recommended, but we had to give it no power over us and that meant we must both have no fear over its arrival. "It" would be gone again soon. Thoughtfully, Tom nodded; he smiled at me and I could see the beginnings of a deeper understanding happening within him. How beautiful I felt just then, seeing this light of trust inside Tom, his earlier distress vanished. We knew that the new chemo medication could be disruptive to me in the sense I would slow down a bit, be tired, and have more "off" days, but according to my doctor "maybe not too much." We would just have to wait and see. Dr. Antin and his team had indicated a few times to me that I might not need to stay on the medication for more than a year. The greatest benefit to me is that during the next year, the drug would do the fighting in knocking down the Philadelphia Chromosome, allowing my immune system to finally have a chance to fully and completely recover.

In the following days I began to crave a more solid spiritual answer as to why my leukemia had reappeared, so I once again sought out White Eagle's book *Heal Thyself*. My intuition told me to open to page 22 and right there again I found the paragraph I quoted from earlier in this book about God's promise that "nothing can really touch or hurt" us. But for me right now it is the first paragraph on this page that is noteworthy for me to study again. The title of the chapter is **"Creative Thought,"** and the paragraph reads:

> Remember, brethren, what we have told you of
> the cause of disease and the source of all healing;
> remember also that your habitual thoughts
> either create or destroy. Lack of harmony in your

thoughts or in your life brings disease; harmony brings health. Therefore let go all resentment, fear and criticism. Hold only the positive thought of all-good, God, and light will flow into you.

And so with these simple but deeply significant words to guide me I will embrace deeper into my soul what is needed for me to do regarding my past. I must surrender ... trust and without fear – *LET GO!*

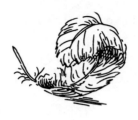

Michael

M Y YOUNGEST BROTHER MICHAEL IS A VERY WISE SOUL. HE
walks on this earth lightly and without excess baggage, his greatest wish – to find a loving mate to
spend his remaining days with. Michael is a healer, a spirit
whose greatest personal truth is that he lives his life in truth.
Michael is not without his personal pain nor is he without
his doubts and fears. But he *knows* that he is a spiritual
being here on Earth living a journey to *remember.*

As I complete this work now I recall a poem that I read
many years ago when I first began to search for spiritual
truths and answers in life. It was a beautiful piece about the
Lord calling a fearful soul to come to the edge of the mountain. The soul responded to the Lord that he was afraid.

The Lord asked softly for the soul to trust and to come closer to the edge of the mountain. The soul began walking forward slowly, but with eyes squeezed shut. The Lord asked tenderly for the soul to open his eyes, to stand at the edge of the mountain and be unafraid ... to leap into the air ... and to trust! The soul said he could not, but ... with a gentle nudge from the Lord, the soul fell off the safety of the mountain ... *and* HE FLEW!

May love and light be yours forever.

I Promise

It's funny how a whole world can change in a day
A minute
A second
Funny how a whole world can change
From a sentence
Maybe a word
It's funny when death is no longer a distant promise,
But a present threat
It's funny how everything you knew you had —
Or didn't know you had —
Everything that gave you meaning,
Gave you life,
Is gone.
Maybe just for now.
But maybe forever.
It's funny how we have a choice —
Effective immediately —
Run and hide?
Run towards it with fists flying?
Stand steady and see what happens?
It's funny what that choice says about people
It's funny when the one in pain is stronger

Than the one watching the pain
It's funny how sometimes it hurts more
To love someone in pain
Than to be in pain.
It's funny how we can grow up in a matter of
Weeks
Days
Maybe seconds.
It's funny that we have to say it's funny because we
    know that we can either
Laugh or cry.
It's funny how laughter in the midst of pain is strong,
    beautiful, and powerful
It's funny how we say everything is gonna be ok
It's funny how we discover faith, hope, determination,
    desperation
That we never knew we had,
With those words.
Everything's gonna be ok
Everything is gonna be ok
I promise

Emily Kane

Emily is a sixteen-year-old girl whose mother, a patient at Dana Farber, is undergoing treatment for acute leukemia. Emily was kind enough to grant us permission to reprint I Promise here.